VASCULAR MECHANISMS OF THE BRAIN

G. I. Mchedlishvili

Institute of Physiology
Georgian Academy of Sciences
Tbilisi, USSR

Translated from Russian

CONSULTANTS BUREAU • NEW YORK—LONDON • 1972

The Russian text, originally published by Nauka Press in Leningrad in 1968, has been extensively revised and corrected by the author for this edition. The present translation is published under an agreement with Mezhdunarodnaya Kniga, the Soviet book export agency.

Г. И. МЧЕДЛИШВИЛИ

ФУНКЦИЯ СОСУДИСТЫХ МЕХАНИЗМОВ ГОЛОВНОГО МОЗГА

Library of Congress Catalog Card Number 70-141241

ISBN 0-306-10870-4

A Division of Plenum Publishing Corporation
227 West 17th Street, New York, N. Y. 10011

United Kingdom edition published by Consultants Bureau, London
A Division of Plenum Publishing Company, Ltd.
Davis House (4th Floor), 8 Scrubs Lane, Harlesden, NW10 6SE, London, England

Printed in the United States of America

PREFACE

The author of this book began his research into the normal and pathological physiology of the circulation in the 1940s. This research followed two main lines: to begin with it was devoted to general problems of the microcirculation, generalized in the monograph "The Capillary Circulation" (Georgian Academy of Sciences, Tbilisi, 1958), while later it was concerned with the regulation and disturbances of the cerebral circulation. Ten years of experimental research in this field on animals yielded much new information of considerable interest both to investigators working in the field of the regional circulation and microcirculation, and also to physicians meeting with cerebrovascular distrubances in their daily practice. The first general account of these investigations was given in the monograph "Function of the Vascular Mechanisms of the Brain" (Nauka, Leningrad, 1968). Although only a few years have elapsed since the publication of that book, much experimental material has been collected in the intervening period, with the result that the contents and arrangement of some of the chapters must be modified for the second edition, and new results of research and new bibliographic references added.

The first stage of this research into the cerebral circulation was undertaken in the laboratory directed by the eminent Soviet pathophysiologist and honorary member of the Georgian Academy of Sciences Professor V. V. Voronin, who until 1960 was head of the Department of Pathological Physiology and Morphology at the Institute of Physiology of the Georgian Academy of Sciences. This Institute was founded and the whole of its activity has been constantly directed by Professor I. S. Beritashvili, Academician of the Academy of Sciences of the USSR, the Academy of Medical Sciences of the USSR, and the Georgian Academy of Sciences. The scientific stmosphere of this Institute and the daily contacts with the workers in its laboratories went a long way toward ensuring the success of the research.

The results of investigations of the cerebral circulation conducted in the author's laboratory and described in this book could never have been obtained without the tremendous efforts of all its staff, as well as those of specialists from the Institute of Physiology, Georgian Academy of Sciences and other scientific institutions in Tbilisi who have collaborated with me. Among these I should like to mention especially R. V. Antia, D. G. Baramidze, N. P. Mitagvaria, L. S. Nikolaishvili and L. G. Ormotsadze (Department of Pathophysiology and Morphology of this Institute), G. V. Amashukeli (Georgian Postgraduate Medical Institute), V. A. Akhobadze (M. D. Tsinamzgvrishvili Institute of Experimental and Clinical Cardiology, Ministry of Health of the Georgian SSR), V. M. Gabashvili and M. G. Devdariani (Institute of Clinical and Experimental Neurology, Ministry of Health of the Georgian SSR), P. A. Kometiani and V. N. Chikvaidze (Department of Biochemistry of the Institute of Physiology, Georgian Academy of Sciences) and A. I. Roitbak (Laboratory of General Physiology of the Cerebral Cortex of that Institute). An important part in the investigations was played by joint work with scientists abroad and in other cities of the USSR: E. K. Plechkova, N. B. Lavrent'eva, O. Ya. Kaufman and A. V. Borodula (Institute of Normal and Pathological Physiology, Academy of Medical Sciences of the USSR, Moscow), V. M. Samvelian (Institute of Cardiology and Heart Surgery, Ministry of Health of the Armenian SSR, Erevan), T. Garbulinski and A. Gosk (Wroclaw, Poland), and also with D. Ingvar, C. Owman, B. Falck and R. Ekberg (Lund, Sweden). I take this opportunity of expressing my sincere thanks to all of them.

The author is deeply grateful to all his colleagues and friends who, by their friendly advice and critical comments, have assisted him with these investigations of the cerebral circulation and with the preparation of this book for publication.

The author hopes that this book will promote

further experimental research into the physiology and pathology of the cerebral circulation and that it will also prove useful to the practicing physician. If this hope is even partly fulfilled, he will be able to rest assured that the long and sustained work of himself and his colleagues will not have been in vain.

Professor George Mchedlishvili, M.D.,
Department of Pathophysiology
Institute of Physiology
Georgian Academy of Sciences,
Tbilisi, USSR

CONTENTS

PART 2
PHYSIOLOGICAL MECHANISMS OF FUNCTIONAL BEHAVIOR OF THE CEREBRAL ARTERIES

INTRODUCTION

The brain certainly needs a more constant and better regulated blood supply than any other of the body. The blood flow through a human brain weighing 1400 g (approximately 2% of the body weight) is about 750 ml/min, i.e., approximately 15-20% of all blood expelled by the heart into the systemic circulation passes through the brain per minute [143]. In 1 min the brain utilizes on the average 49 ml of oxygen, i.e., about 20% of the total quantity utilized by all tissues of the body [365], and 76 ml glucose, i.e., 70% of all the glucose issuing from the liver [340]. Under normal conditions the principal source of energy needed for neuron function is oxidation of glucose. However, the brain has no reserve of carbohydrates, and still less of oxygen, so that its normal metabolism depends entirely on a constant supply of blood-borne energy-giving materials. If the circulation stops, severe metabolic disturbances at once arise in the brain. The high sensitivity of the brain to disturbances of its blood supply, on the one hand, and the comparative vulnerability of its vascular system, on the other hand, explain why changes in brain function are most frequently dependent on circulatory disorders. Such changes include headaches, disturbances of ability to do intellectual work, loss of memory in elderly people; and a great variety of neurological disorders caused by brain trauma, apoplexy, etc. could be mentioned. During circulatory deficiency not all brain functions are equally sensitive, of course, to oxygen lack: speech and intellectual activity are the first to be disturbed, loss of consciousness takes place 5-6 sec after complete interruption of the circulation, and death ensues after 4-5 min [340].

Progress in practical medicine, so far as the development and effects of cerebrovascular disturbances are concerned, is primarily dependent on experimental investigations of the cerebral circulation under normal and pathological conditions. Without them it would be impossible to understand which vascular responses and circulatory phenomena are harmful or unsuited to brain activity and which, on the contrary, are compensatory or protective in character. It is only by thorough analysis of the physiological principles governing these phenomena that the physician, when he attempts to interfere with the processes taking place in the body, can be confident that he is doing good, and not harm, to the patient.

The history of investigations of the physiology of the cerebral circulation has passed through several periods. a) The first, which lasted until the end of the 19th century, was dominated by the Monro–Kellie doctrine [278, 140]. Proceeding from the assumption that the skull is rigid and its contents incompressible, it was thought that the blood volume and circulation in the brain must remain fixed whatever the conditions. b) After the appearance of Leonard Hill's classical monograph [111] a new concept came to be accepted: the cerebral circulation may vary but only by the operation of an extrinsic mechanism, i.e., through changes in the systemic arterial pressure, and not by vasomotor responses of the cerebral blood vessels; the principal postulate of the Monro–Kellie doctrine, that the blood volume within the skull remains constant, was thus still accepted. This concept was held almost universally until the 1930s. c) With the gradual accumulation of experimental data, evidence was obtained for the important role of an intrinsic mechanism, i.e., of the vasomotor responses of the cerebral arteries, in the control of blood supply to the brain. This concept was summarized in a number of publications which appeared in the 1950s [341, 148, 170, 367, 175].

Since in most of the investigations to that period all that had been done was to record the blood flow or the resistance in the vascular system of the brain, the results could not possibly show how the different vessels of the brain participate in regulation and in disturbances of the regional circulation. It was therefore necessary to assume that either regulation of the local hemodynamics in the brain is effected by the "cerebral vessels" (without specifying which vessels), or, alternatively, the leading role was ascribed to the "arterioles." Although originally the term "arterioles" had the concrete meaning of the smallest precapillary arteries, the walls of which contain a single layer of muscle cells, later on it was applied to all small arteries (down to 300-500 μ in caliber) capable of changing their lumen within wide limits.

By the end of the 1950s a new problem had arisen. It was necessary to elucidate the general principles governing the functional behavior of the intrinsic mechanisms regulating the cerebral circulation and concerned in its disorders. This problem was closely related to those engaging the attention of researchers in the microcirculation field. To study differences in the functional behavior of different parts of the vascular system of the brain and, in particular, differences in their responses to nervous and humoral influences, their role in regulating the blood supply to the brain, in compensating cerebrovascular disorders, and in the genesis of circulatory disturbances in the central nervous system, it was essential that the research methods used should yield, not indirect data, but concrete and quantitative information concerning the functional behavior of each part of the vascular system of the brain, and especially of its arterial system. It is well known that in the vascular system of every organ, the principal "controllable" component is the capillary circulation, and the most active "controlling" part the arterial vessels. The intensity of the capillary circulation and all its changes under normal and pathological conditions are dependent on the total resistance of the whole extent of the arterial system of the organ, starting from the main arteries as they enter the organ (branches of the central arteries, the pressure in which is regarded as the systemic arterial pressure), and ending with the tiny precapillary arterioles. At a given moment, depending on the concrete conditions, one or another part of the arterial system of any organ may change its lumen like a valve, and thus bring about appropriate changes in the capillary circulation. The author's investigations into the mechanisms of the microcirculation [208] have demonstrated that the intrinsic arteries of an organ play an important role in modifying many aspects of the capillary circulation: the velocity of the blood flow in the capillaries, the distribution of blood cells in capillary networks, changes in the number of active capillaries, the onset and compensation of disturbances of the capillary circulation, such as intracapillary aggregation of erythrocytes, the complex group of circulatory changes in an inflammatory focus, and so on.

The concept of a distinctive role of different parts of the arterial system of organs was concisely formulated by Voronin [397], who concluded from experimental results obtained in his laboratory [28, 396, 409] that the larger arteries of organs (those possessing a well-developed muscular layer) are directly concerned with regulation of the systemic arterial pressure, while the smaller arteries regulate the blood supply of the tissue in accordance with its metabolic needs. These researches were continued by Voronin's co-workers: the present author studied the cerebral circulation, other workers [91] studied the functional peculiarities of the skin arteries, and so on.

Until recently very few experimental data concerning the functional behavior of different parts of the vascular system of the brain had been published. The most likely explanations of this fact are, first, that the problem was simply not considered by the overwhelming majority of investigators and, second, the usual approaches and methods could not elucidate the peculiarities of the functional behavior of different parts of the cerebrovascular system. The characteristic physiological behavior of blood vessels regulating the cerebral circulation could be found out under the conditions either when they correlate the blood supply with changes in brain function under physiological conditions or when compensation of cerebrovascular disturbances takes place under pathological conditions. The study of the functional behavior of the vascular mechanisms under pathological conditions appeared to the author to be most promising, for these conditions are extremely varied and, consequently, many different types of functional behavior of different parts of the cerebrovascular system are available for study; moreover, under pathological conditions the changes may be much more marked quantitatively and, therefore, more easily detectable than under physiological conditions.

At the very outset of the author's investigations of the cerebral circulation (in 1956-1957) the active role of the major arteries of the brain in regulating the cerebral blood supply was discovered quite unexpectedly: in a study of cortical capillaries during venous stagnation it was found that intravital fixation of the cortex with excision of part of the hemispheres (for microscopic investigation) immediately after occlusion of the jugular veins was accompanied by unexpectedly slight bleeding. The gradual accumulation of experimental data eventually showed that under these conditions venous stagnation is not present in the brain. It was later discovered that this is because of constriction of the whole system of major arteries of the brain, and that it is a compensatory reaction, i.e., a manifestation of regulation of the cerebral circulation. The regulatory role of the major arteries of the brain was subsequently demonstrated under different conditions. It was soon found that responses (constriction or dilatation) of individual vessels throughout the arterial system cannot only differ in degree, but also be opposite in direction. This compelled the introduction of a new concept of "vascular mechanism," implying a combination of functional properties of a given vessel or vessels, or in other words, those features of the structure and function of the vessel walls which determine their responses to various stimuli, together with the stimuli (nervous, humoral, or other) which control the size of the lumen and, consequently, the resistance in these vessels. From the author's point of view, those parts of a blood vessel which, throughout their extent, exhibit relatively uniform functional properties and give identical responses to various stimuli, can be regarded as a separate vascular mechanism. From work done during the 1960s, it has become apparent that functional behavior may differ in the following parts of the cerebrovascular system: a) the major arteries of the brain* (the internal carotid and vertebral arteries), b) the pial arteries (the intermediate segments between the pial and cortical arteries), d) the intracerebral arteries and arterioles, e) the capillaries, f) the pial veins, and g) the emissary veins of the skull carrying blood from the brain sinuses. Very probably with improvements in research methods it will later be possible to differentiate the vascular mechanisms of the brain, from the standpoint of functional behavior, in even greater detail. This may apply to blood vessels of different caliber and also to vessels in different parts of the brain.

The introduction of this new concept of "vascular mechanism" into circulatory physiology was determined by three factors: a) the need to draw a sharp line between parts of the vascular system of an organ with different functions and to study their role in its contribution to its peripheral resistance; b) the need for combined investigation of all the functional properties of these vascular regions; and c) the need to establish the functional organization of the intrinsic mechanisms of regulation and disturbance of the local circulation and microcirculation in each organ. Under present-day conditions, it would be impossible without such an approach to understand the mechanisms regulating the circulation and microcirculation within an organ or to be able to treat their disorders in disease. From this point of view, the vascular system of the brain is in a slightly advantageous position, for in the case of most other organs neither suitable methods of investigation nor experimental results reflecting the functional behavior of the various vascular mechanisms are yet available.

Since this book is devoted only to one particular aspect of investigation of the cerebral circulation, which has been widely developed in the laboratory directed by its author, the reader will find that it contains principally experimental data emanating from that laboratory, and that it does not attempt to give an exhaustive account of the history of research in the field of the physiology and pathology of the cerebral circulation in general.

*In a number of papers written by the author these arteries were called "regional arteries of the brain," because in Voronin's laboratories the term "regional arteries" was used to describe all arteries of medium caliber and of muscular type entering an organ and playing an important role in the creation of peripheral resistance. Later, however, the use of this term led to difficulties because the word "regional" literally means "local" when applied to arteries, and many writers use this term to describe all the arteries of an organ, of whatever type.

PART 1

FUNCTIONAL BEHAVIOR OF THE VASCULAR MECHANISMS OF THE BRAIN UNDER VARIOUS CONDITIONS

CHAPTER I

INVESTIGATING THE BEHAVIOR OF DIFFERENT PARTS OF THE CEREBROVASCULAR SYSTEM

The hemodynamics of the brain is, to a large extent, determined by the cerebrovascular resistance which is dependent, in its turn, on the functional state of the whole vascular system, starting from the arteries entering the skull and ending with the veins draining blood from the brain. Hence the need for obtaining the fullest information possible concerning the behavior of all portions of the vascular system of the brain under all conditions studied. This is why, in the investigations on which the present book is based, the methods commonly used were those which simultaneously indicated the functional behavior of different parts of its vascular system. If this was impossible, or if the information obtained was insufficient to give a complete picture of behavior of the cerebrovascular system, several series of analogous experiments were carried out with appropriate variation of the parameters studied. When methods of investigation were chosen, attempts were made to ensure that they satisfied the following conditions. First, the methods of investigation to be used must reveal the nature of the studied phenomenon directly, and not simply provide indirect data, sometimes difficult to interpret. Second, the methods used must as far as possible give quantitative results; this is important not merely in connection with estimation of the physiological importance of the results, but also with their subsequent statistical analysis. To study the functional behavior of the various vascular mechanisms of the brain the methods described below were used.

1. The major arteries of the brain, the internal carotid and vertebral arteries, are particularly difficult to investigate because much of their course lies inside bony canals and within the venous sinuses, in which they are inaccessible for direct intravital observation. Investigations on mammals were facilitated a little by the fact that the major arteries of the brain, being connected together in the region of the circle of Willis by wide arterial anastomoses, constitute a single functional system (Chapter V). In some cases, in order to obtain continuous recordings of the functional state of these vessels, one of the carotid arteries had to be excluded from the circulation, but because of the existence of these wide anastomoses in the region of the circle of Willis, this procedure should not significantly disturb the blood supply to the brain [141, 40, 103]. The following methods were used to investigate the functional state of the major arteries of the brain.

A. By recording the rate of outflow of blood from the circle of Willis through the internal carotid artery, for example, by means of a drop counter, with a stabilized aortic pressure, dynamic determinations could be made of the resistance in the following portions of the vascular system: the three active major arteries of the brain, the circle of Willis, and the isolated internal carotid artery. This technique was used only at the very beginning of the author's studies in the field – at the end of the 1950s. To avoid mistakes in interpretation, allowance had also to be made for the resistance in the cerebral vessels peripherally to the circle of Willis. However, as happened when this resistance was obviously increased, e.g., when all the jugular veins in the neck were excluded and the pial arteries constricted, a decrease in the outflow of blood from the circle of Willis through one of the internal carotid arteries must have indicated an increase in resistance in the system of the major arteries of the brain [209].

B. By measuring the blood pressure simultaneously in the aorta and in the circle of Willis, the pressure gradient can be estimated along the major arteries of the brain to judge the resistance in them [211, 219]. By means of a catheter introduced into one of the common carotid arteries in the direction of the thorax, the blood pressure was recorded in the aorta and in its major branches, i.e., at the origin of the other three major arteries of the brain (the other carotid artery and the vertebral arteries); a second catheter, introduced in the cranial direction, recorded the blood pressure in the circle of Willis. All branches of this carotid artery in the rabbits and dogs were preliminarily ligated, except the internal carotid artery as a result of which the artery acted as a continuation of the catheter and connected it directly to the circle of Willis (Fig. 1).

In dogs additional anastomoses exist between the internal and external carotid arteries (or more accurately, the branches of the external carotid: the external orbital and middle meningeal arteries). The operative approach to the anastomosis connecting the internal carotid artery and the external orbital artery, a branch of the maxillary artery, in the dog has been perfected by several investigators [25, 337, 380]. In the writer's experiments, the skin incision was made along the sagittal line beneath the lower jaw and was then carried deep between the digastric and mylohyoid muscles as far as the pterygoid muscle. The pterygoid muscle was detached from bone by diathermy knife, and retracted laterally, thus opening up the access to the maxillary artery. This vessel was carefully dissected toward the periphery as far as the external orbital artery, and the anastomosis was then identified. A ligature was applied to the anastomosis, or if this

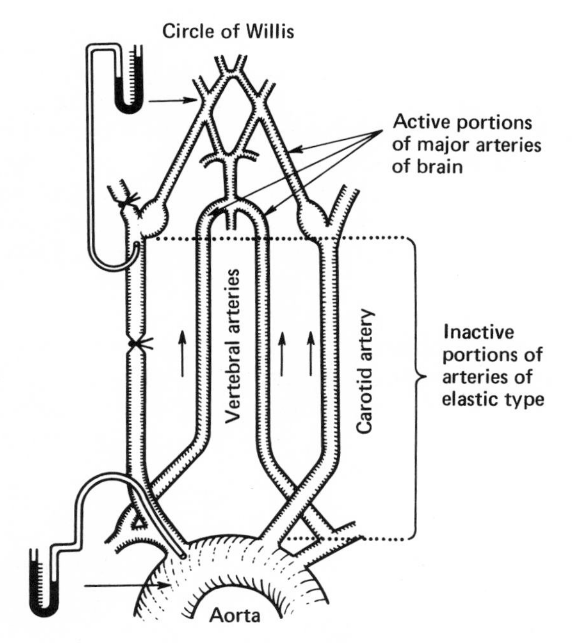

Fig. 1. Scheme of determination of resistance along the major arteries of the brain on the basis of pressure differences in the aorta and circle of Willis. Explanation in text.

was impossible, it was coagulated and dissected. Since the middle meningeal artery leaves the maxillary artery inside the pterygoid canal, the latter vessel was ligated at its entrance to and exit from this canal, thus excluding the middle meningeal artery. A control injection of contrast material into the internal carotid artery after the experiment showed conclusively that all its branches had been excluded. The experiment showed that exclusion of all the anastomoses causes only a slight increase (of a few millimeters of mercury) in the pressure recorded in the circle of Willis.*

The pressure gradient in the system of major arteries of the brain, from the aorta as far as the circle of Willis, enables an estimate to be made of changes in the resistance of the internal carotid and vertebral arteries only under the following conditions: a) if the systemic arterial pressure remains constant (if necessary it can be stabilized artificially by means of a compensator – see below); b) if there are no primary and well-marked changes in the velocity of blood flow in the major arteries of the brain, as occur, for example, after exclusion of the cranial vena cava [232], when the reduction of the pressure gradient in the major arteries of the brain gives no indication of their dilatation (p. 69); c) if there are no significant changes in resistance of the cerebral arteries located peripherally to the circle of Willis. For example, when the pial arteries were widely dilated (in asphyxia and in postischemic states of the brain), one could not be certain that an increase in the pressure gradient in the major arteries of the brain actually reflected their constriction, and other methods of investigation had to be used, namely, recording the volume velocity of the blood flow in them, [241, 332] or resistography of the isolated internal carotid artery *in situ* (see below).

C. By recording the blood flow in the internal carotid arteries by means of any type of flowmeter, changes in the lumen of these arteries can be estimated [332, 242, 90, 241]. However, under these circumstances allowance had to be made for changes in the systemic arterial pressure (if necessary this can be stabilized artificially), and the state of the pial, precortical, and intracerebral vessels must also be taken into consideration. Finally, the blood flow in the internal carotid artery

*When all anastomoses are intact, blood evidently flows along them into branches of the external carotid artery, which was ligated in these experiments at its mouth. The difference between the manometer readings reflects the resistance from the circle of Willis to the mouth of the anastomosis.

reflected the state of its lumen in cases when, during local manipulations of the vessel, the blood flow in the contralateral internal carotid artery was unchanged, for extensive anastomoses in the region of the circle of Willis ensure equalization of the blood pressure at the end of both internal carotid arteries. When experiments were carried out on dogs, it was important to exclude all anastomoses between the internal and branches of the external carotid arteries, because it has been known for a long time that after ligation of the external carotid artery (which is always done in these experiments) most of the blood flows out through these anastomoses into its peripheral branches [33], and for this reason the flowmeter readings always reflect the state of both the active parts of the internal carotid artery and of extracranial branches of different caliber. In experiments on dogs, all connections must therefore be abolished between the internal and external carotid arteries (the operation is described above).

D. A method of measuring resistance in the isolated internal carotid artery *in situ*, recently developed, has been used in two modifications. In the first [257], a constant volume of blood is injected from the common carotid artery, by a perfusion pump with constant minute volume, into the internal carotid artery, which is left *in situ*, but has all its connections with the extracerebral vessels excluded, and after the blood has entered the intracranial cavity it flows from it via a thin polyethylene tube directly into the jugular vein. The changes in perfusion pressure in these experiments thus reflected the vascular resistance in the internal carotid artery only.*

The catheter of a perfusion pump was inserted into the cranial end of the ligated common carotid artery, all branches of which, except the internal carotid artery, were ligated. All anastomoses between the internal carotid and external orbital arteries, and also the middle meningeal artery (see above), had to be ligated in dogs. To introduce another catheter into the internal carotid artery inside the skull, the operative approach to the base of the brain was made through the temporal bone. The skull was widely trephined, the dura opened, and the brain gradually displaced with a spatula superiorly and caudally, until the circle of Willis was reached. The anterior cerebral and posterior communicating arteries were ligated at their origins. A polyethylene catheter was introduced into the middle cere-

*This experimental technique may be modified as follows. Instead of recording the perfusion pressure, the volume velocity of the blood flow can also be measured continuously by means of any type of flowmeter, but under these circumstances the level of the systemic arterial pressure must remain constant.

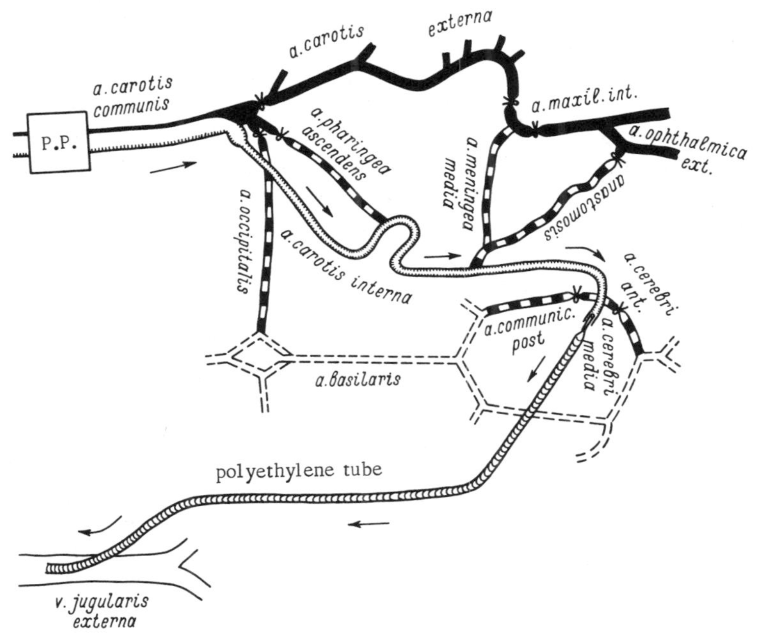

Fig. 2. Scheme of hemodynamic isolation of internal carotid artery in dogs [257, 259]. Explanation in text. The vessels in which blood is circulating are shown in white, system of external carotid artery shown in black, ligated branches of internal carotid artery shown in black and white. Arrows indicate direction of blood flow. P.P., perfusion pump.

bral artery, its end reaching as far as the mouth of the internal carotid artery. The catheter was connected by a polyethylene tube to the animal's external jugular vein. In this way it was possible to perfuse only the internal carotid artery, from which blood was carried directly into the venous system, by-passing the smaller cerebral vessels (Fig. 2). When the experiments were carried out in this way, the vessel, which was continuously perfused with blood, remained *in situ* and all its nervous connections were intact, i.e., the experimental conditions were as close to natural as possible. Under relatively superficial anesthesia, the walls of the internal carotid arteries reacted to small doses of physiologically active substances and to other agents and the resistance in the vessel was modified within wide limits, even to the extent of complete functional occlusion of its lumen for varied periods of time.

Provided that certain conditions are observed, resistography of the isolated internal carotid artery *in situ* can evidently also be carried out with the vessels of the circle of Willis intact. This is possible because the four major arteries of the brain are joined together both at their beginning (aorta) and at their end (circle of Willis) and the wide arterial anastomoses in the region of the circle of Willis ensure equalization of pressure in all its parts. The magnitude of the perfusion pressure in the internal carotid artery thus reflects the resistance in this vessel only under the following conditions. First, when the level of the systemic arterial pressure and, consequently, of the pressure in the circle of Willis, remains stable throughout the experiment, for example, during injection of minimal doses of physiologically active substances such as noradrenalin or acetylcholine into the investigated artery. Second, an increase in perfusion pressure reflects an increase in resistance in the internal carotid artery when the pressure in the circle of Willis falls as a result of a fall of the systemic arterial pressure, or for other reasons, for example, in terminal states or in the last stages of asphyxia. In this modification of measurement of the perfusion pressure in the internal carotid artery, just as in the method described above, all anastomoses connecting this vessel with the extracerebral arteries must be excluded. The writer's experiments have shown that characteristic responses of the internal carotid arteries appear under widely different conditions.

E. In the second method of resistography of the isolated internal carotid artery *in situ* [256], this artery, isolated in a dog as described above, was perfused from a reservoir of oxygenated Ringer's bicarbonate solution, heated to body temperature, of the following composition: NaCl 0.69%, KCl 0.035%, $CaCl_2$ 0.028%, KH_2PO_4 0.16%, $MgSO_4 \cdot 7H_2O$ 0.029%, $NaHCO_3$ 0.21%, and glucose 0.05%; pH 7.4. This perfusion fluid was injected into the artery by means of a pump with constant minute volume, so that the perfusion pressure reflected the resistance in the internal carotid artery only (Fig. 3). Despite the fact that the perfusion fluid used was free from colloids and, consequently, did not possess a colloid-osmotic pressure, perfusion of the internal carotid artery with it for 5-6 h during a short-term experiment did not result in significant edema of the vessel wall, for no persistent increase of resistance in the vessel calling for administration of spasmolytic drugs of the papaverine type was usually observed in the course of the experiment. Throughout this period the artery remained highly sensitive to physiologically active substances and, in particular, to serotonin.

In contrast to methods widely used to analyze the function of arterial walls *in vitro*, on excised strips of vessel walls (mainly the largest arteries such as the aorta and its branches, which do not participate in the regulation of vascular resistance in general or of the blood supply of organs in particular), the present method has the following advantages: it studies the functional behavior of the wall of a particular vessel (the internal carotid artery), playing an important role in regulating the inflow of blood into the brain, actually *in situ*; the constant-volume perfusion pump ensures stable conditions of perfusion of the blood vessel which can be varied at will; unlimited opportunities exist

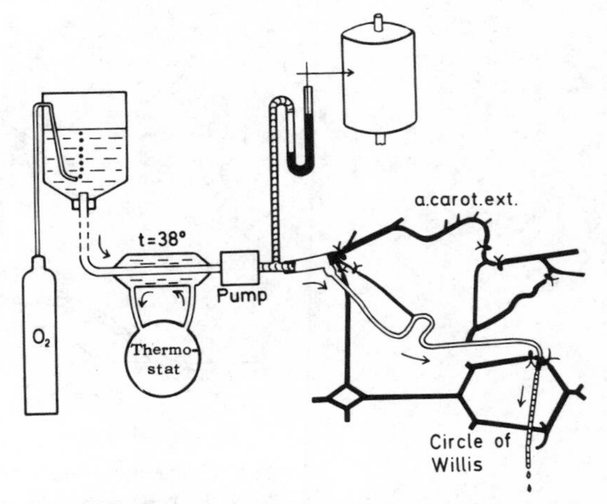

Fig. 3. Second method of resistography of the isolated internal carotid artery of a dog *in situ* [256]. Explanation in text.

for changing the composition of the perfusion fluid, and any excess of substances injected are eliminated from the body. Consequently, this method satisfies the optimal requirements for investigations of this type [83].

F. Determination of resistance in the major arteries of the brain and also in smaller arteries lying peripherally to the circle of Willis, using an adequate mathematical model [248,276]. Having regard to the specific conditions of this approach, besides certain simplifications in the structure of the system regulating the cerebral circulation, the following assumptions were also permitted: a) constancy of the relative viscosity of the blood and b) changes in the resistance to the blood flow only during active changes in lumen of the vessels. Subsequent tests showed that these assumptions evidently did not significantly affect the adequacy of the experimental model. The original data for construction of the mathematical model were obtained in experiments on preparations of the isolated internal carotid artery of dogs, in which the vessel was left in a piece of bone with its geometrical shape intact, and was perfused either with saline or blood plasma from a reservoir or with blood from the arterial system of a donor dog. By recording the pressure at the inlet and outlet of the artery and measuring the volume velocity of flow of the liquid (blood), and by artificially changing the resistance in various segments of the artery quantitative characteristics were obtained to describe the relationship between these parameters. By mathematical analysis of the results using a computer, a regression equation of the following form was obtained:

$$P_{cW}/P_a = a_0 + a_1R_m + a_2R_p + a_3R_mR_p + a_4R_m^2 + a_5R_p^2 + a_6R_m^3 + a_7R_p^3 \qquad (1)$$

where P_{cW} is the pressure in the circle of Willis, P_a the pressure in the aorta, R_m the resistance in the major arteries of the brain, and R_p the resistance in the brain vessels located peripherally to the circle of Willis. Correlation and regression analysis of equation (1) demonstrated its high accuracy.

The second equation, with the same unknowns, described the principle of continuity of circulation of the blood, and as applied to the cerebral circulation it could be written in the following form:

$$\frac{P_a - P_{cW}}{R_m} = \frac{P_{cW} - P_c}{R_p} \qquad (2)$$

where P_c is the pressure in the venous sinuses of the brain, and the remaining symbols have the same meaning as in equation (1). Equation (2) establishes the equality of the volume velocities of blood flow through the major arteries and corresponding small arteries of the brain located peripherally to the circle of Willis.

Comparison of the results of direct experimental measurements and those calculated from the model demonstrated its high adequacy ($R = 0.96$). Hence, having once obtained an adequate mathematical model, and using the pressures recorded in the aorta, the circle of Willis, and the venous sinuses of the brain in physiological experiments, it was possible to investigate with an electronic computer, and under different experimental conditions, the dynamics of changes in resistance in the major arteries of the brain and also in the small arteries located peripherally to the circle of Willis.

The reasons for the wide variety of methods listed above for the investigation of functional behavior of the major arteries of the brain are, first, the difficulty of obtaining direct and quantitative data concerning the width of these arteries (with the one exception of investigation of the isolated internal carotid arteries *in situ*) and second, the fact that in most cases the results obtained reflected the state of these arteries only under particular conditions. It therefore became necessary in some cases to use several methods as a cross check on the conclusion regarding the state of the major arteries of the brain under particular conditions.

2. The pial arteries, located on the brain surface, are accessible to direct observation if the skull is trephined and the dura removed. If a plastic "window" is inserted into the cranial bones, the intracranial pressure is prevented from falling, although the writer has observed that this factor is not as important as many researchers are inclined to believe (probably as a legacy from the Monro–Kellie doctrine). There may even be advantages in studying the pial arteries under open skull conditions because they remain under steady extravascular pressure throughout the experiment. Under the microscope, the pial arteries can be clearly distinguished against the pale background of the brain surface. However, direct measurements of their diameter with the ocular micrometer are difficult because of the mobility of the object and of the fact that it is impossible to measure the width of several vessels at the same time. Serial microfilming has therefore been carried out by the author and his co-workers at intervals of 5-10 sec and the time of each photograph indicated

on the recording paper (microcinematography would have been useless, since the responses of the pial arteries are comparatively slow under different conditions). During microphotography the brain surface was illuminated with "cold" light from a mercury–quartz lamp (for example, the OI-18), with a filter cutting out ultraviolet rays. Measurements of the diameter of chosen arteries under the microscope were made with the aid of an ocular micrometer on each frame of the film (during printing on photographic paper, distortions may arise depending on the length of exposure). To make the results more conclusive, the person measuring the vascular diameter did not know to what stage of the experiment a particular frame pertained. By plotting the results on recording paper (together with other parameters) a curve illustrating the whole dynamics of changes in the width of the pial arteries with time was obtained [e.g., 212, 213, 214].

The ratio between the volume of erythrocytes and plasma in the pial arteries can be investigated in relation to various changes in the cerebral circulation [216, 240]. The vessels were fixed *in situ* on the brain surface by means of 20% formalin in 96° ethanol, and total microscopic preparations were made of the pia mater. To determine the content of erythrocytes and plasma in the pial arteries, the diameter of the vessels and the width of the axial flow of erythrocytes were measured. The proportion of the lumen of the vessel occupied by erythrocytes and the portion occupied by plasma could then be calculated.

3. The functional behavior of the precortical arteries – short intermediate portions between the pial and radial arteries entering the cortex – was investigated in total preparations of the blood vessels in the pia fixed intravitally at the essential stage of the experiment [236]. For this purpose the vascular system of the brain was perfused under standard conditions (appropriate to the experiment) with a fixing fluid of the following composition: 6% formalin made up in a mixture of equal parts 0.85% sodium chloride and 96° ethyl alcohol. This fluid was infused through a catheter, previously inserted in the direction of the internal carotid artery, at the same time as blood was withdrawn from the aorta and while the second common carotid artery was occluded. The animal died immediately after injection of the fixing fluid. After removal of the brain and its further fixation for several days, under a binocular microscope the pia containing all branches of the pial arteries, the intermediate portions between them and the radial arteries, and the initial segments of the radial arteries themselves, up to 100-150 μ in length, was removed carefully from it. The following parameters of the precortical arteries could be determined in these total preparations when examined under the microscope either unstained or stained with hematoxylin-eosin and Van Gieson's method: a) the total length of the vessels from the point of their branching from the pial vessels to their entry into the brain, b) the caliber of the vessels, i.e., the external diameter of their initial portions, c) the external diameter, thickness of the wall, and diameter of the lumen of different portions of the vessel, and d) the length and diameter of nuclei of smooth-muscle cells in the vessel walls. All values obtained under the influence of the various procedures in the experimental animals were compared with those in the controls whose precortical arteries had been fixed in the same way, but without exposure to the corresponding experimental procedures.

4. The functional state of the smaller blood vessels located inside the brain substance, especially arteries, arterioles, and capillaries of the cerebral cortex, was investigated by the method used with other organs in previous studies [205, 382, 370]: in microscopic sections and total preparations after intravital fixation of the brain tissue and of the blood vessels in it at the required moment of the experiment. Initially the cortex was fixed intravitally *in situ* from the surface with 20% formalin in ethanol; the cortex was then excised and treated histologically. The number of capillaries filled with blood was counted and their diameter was measured in transverse microscopic sections through the cortex [206, 216]. In this way the number of active capillaries was determined in the presence of various changes in the cerebral circulation. Later, intravital fixation of the blood vessel walls was carried out from within the lumen of the vessels, by perfusing the brain vessels at the required moment of the experiment with fixing fluid [234, 11, 259]. The experiments were carried out on unanesthetized rabbits, and operations were performed under local procaine anesthesia. A catheter was inserted in the cranial direction into the common carotid artery, and through it, fixing fluid was injected into the internal carotid artery (all other branches having been ligated) under controlled pressure (using a system of the blood pressure compensator type for this purpose – see below); the pressure was about equal to the natural blood pressure in the cerebral vessels. The composition of the fixing fluid was so chosen that it caused no changes (in rabbits) in the

structure of the blood vessel walls: 6% formalin made up in 0.85% sodium chloride solution mixed with an equal volume of 96° ethanol. After injection of the fixing fluid, which immediately killed the animal, the whole brain was immersed in the same solution until next day, after which it was placed for three days in 12% formalin solution in 0.85% sodium chloride solution (without alcohol). The brain was cut into sections on a freezing microtome so that the radial arteries in the sections could be seen throughout the depth of the cortex, or total preparations were made, as mentioned above (p. 12). Blood vessels of the cerebral cortex were then investigated microscopically in unstained sections in which all structural elements of the walls of the arteries, capillaries, and veins were clearly visible because of differences in their refractive index [e.g., 259,244]. The external and internal diameters of the cortical arteries were measured throughout their extent, every 20 μ by means of an ocular micrometer. The blood vessels of other rabbits, each of whose brain was treated and perfused under analogous conditions but none of which was subjected to the experimental procedures, were used as the control. The results were analyzed by statistical methods.

5. The diameter of the pial veins (like that of the arteries) were measured on photographic films after serial photomicrography of the brain surface (p. 11) [209, 232]. The venous pressure in the brain sinuses was measured in the unopened skull through one branch of the external jugular vein, which communicates through a large emissary vein with the transverse venous sinus; all other branches of this vein were ligated. An operation for the ligation of these branches was devised for the experiments on rabbits (Fig. 4) [254]; such an operation on dogs has

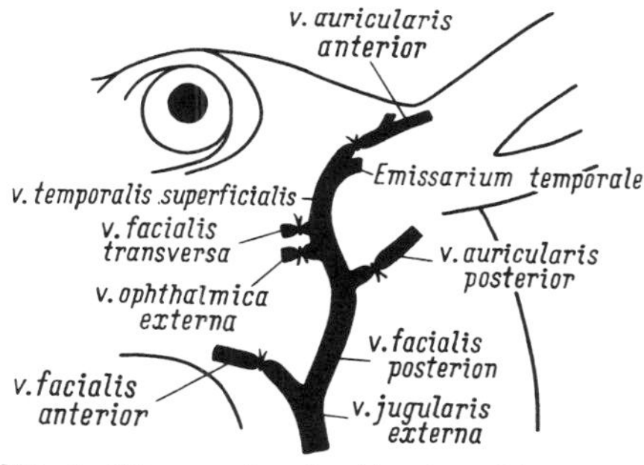

Fig. 4. Diagram showing ligation of branches of the external jugular vein in rabbits to measure pressure in the transverse sinus of the brain without trephining the skull [254].

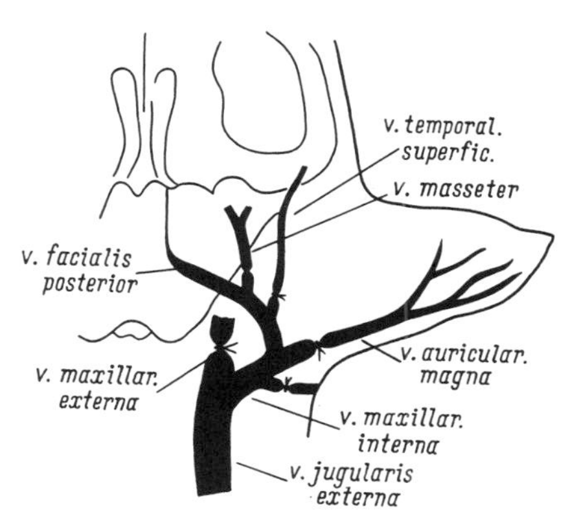

Fig. 5. Diagram showing ligation of branches of external jugular vein in a dog to measure pressure in transverse sinus of brain without trephining the skull [139].

also been performed by other experimenters [118, 139] (Fig. 5). To measure the venous pressure in the sinuses, the polyethylene catheter of a manometer was introduced into the jugular vein in a cranial direction. At the same time, through another catheter introduced through the same jugular vein in the thoracic direction, the blood pressure was measured in the large veins of the thorax. The functional state of the drainage veins carrying blood away from the skull was estimated from the pressure gradient in them, obtained by measuring the pressure simultaneously in the brain sinuses and in the large veins of the thorax [213, 232].

6. Stabilization of the systemic arterial (or venous) pressure was necessary in some cases, since changes in the blood pressure in the aorta (and also in the cranial vena cava) are a factor with considerable effect on the cerebral circulation. The blood pressure compensator consisted of a mercury manometer, a reservoir of air, and a vessel containing blood substitute, connected by means of a wide catheter to one of the large arteries, for example, the femoral artery in dogs or the abdominal aorta below the origin of the renal arteries in rabbits (Fig. 6, II). Pressure in the compensator was kept at the same level as that in the aorta. If the pressure in the aorta rose, blood flowed from the arteries, and if it fell, fluid entered the vessels, as a result of which the blood pressure was automatically and quickly restored to its original level [211]. It was later found to be more convenient to have a reservoir with a relatively large liquid surface, which was kept at the appropriate height (Fig. 6, I). The advantages of this method were, first, that a change in the volume of blood substitute during the experiment had little

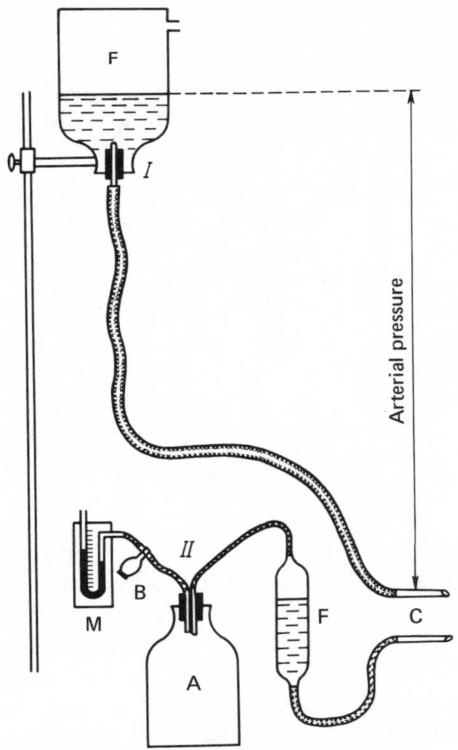

Fig. 6. Diagram showing two types of blood pressure compensator (I and II). Explanation in text. C, catheter introduced into large artery toward the heart; F, blood substitute fluid; A, air reservoir; B, compression bulb with valve; M, manometer measuring pressure in entire system.

effect on the level of its pressure, and second, that this system is more reliable, because the pressure level in it is much more stable (in the system described above, even a very slight leak of air in time changed the pressure level).

Under some conditions such sharp changes in the level of the systemic arterial pressure took place that the blood pressure compensator described above could not control them. To obtain more effective stabilization of the aortic pressure, a thorax–head preparation was developed [217]. All vessels of the abdomen and limbs were excluded from the experimental animal's circulation, i.e., most of the effector mechanisms by means of which the vasomotor centers of the brain can change the level of the systemic arterial pressure were absent (these areas of the vascular system account for a major part of the peripheral resistance and also for changes in the circulating blood volume). In the course of the operation, the subclavian arteries and veins were ligated on both sides at the point where they leave the chest. In addition, the abdominal aorta and caudal vena cava were ligated immediately below the diaphragm. Hence only the vascular system of the chest and head functioned in the animal, and only the following effector mechanisms which could change the level of the aortic pressure were left intact: the heart (changes in the minute blood volume), and the arteries of the head, neck, and chest wall (changes in peripheral resistance). However, the effect of the latter was abolished by the blood pressure compensator, the catheter of which was inserted into the abdominal aorta immediately below the diaphragm (Fig. 7). Experience has shown that rabbits undergoing such operations in most cases survived in a satisfactory functional state for 2-4 h. If the compensator works normally, the aortic pressure remains constant even after injection of, for example, 50-100 μg adrenalin or acetylcholine into the blood stream; and also during strong electrical stimulation of the carotid sinus receptors. The heart–lungs–head preparation possesses some similar features [6, 58]. However, in the writer's opinion, it is less satisfactory than the thorax–head preparation, because it possesses certain disadvantages: the necessity of opening the

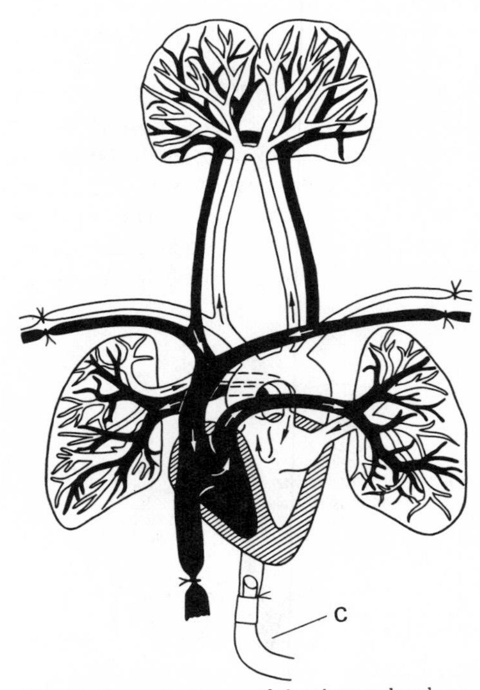

Fig. 7. General scheme of the thorax–head preparation [217]. Explanation in text. C, catheter of blood pressure compensator.

chest and of manipulations in the great vessels located in it; the use of artificial respiration throughout the experiment; the constant circulation of blood through a system of artificial tubes, which may adversely affect the properties of the blood; the absence of automatic stabilization of the aortic pressure.

Other methods which have been used to investigate certain special problems will be mentioned in the appropriate sections of this book.

CHAPTER II

VASCULAR MECHANISMS AND CHANGES IN SYSTEMIC ARTERIAL PRESSURE

It is the systemic arterial pressure that is the basic determining factor of the pressure gradient on which the intensity of the circulation in the intrinsic vessels of all the organs to a great extent depend. The role of the systemic venous pressure level in the pressure gradient is comparatively unimportant, since under ordinary conditions it varies very little (it is only during the action of gravitational forces on the body, e.g., in aviators and astronauts during exposure to high accelerations, that the venous pressure may influence the blood pressure gradient). It is well known that under normal conditions the level of the systemic arterial pressure is kept constant by buffer reflexes, the receptive fields for which are located principally in the arch of the aorta and in the carotid sinus region.

There was a time when any changes in the systemic arterial pressure were thought to produce corresponding changes in the cerebral circulation. This conclusion was drawn by the majority of physiologists from the results of acute animal experiments in which the level of the systemic arterial pressure was raised (e.g., when the pressure in the carotid sinus region was lowered, peripheral nerves were stimulated, etc.). In these cases the constrictor response of arteries in different organs differed in its magnitude; however, the brain arteries (like those of the myocardium) as a rule were not constricted under these circumstances, so that the circulation in them was increased. It was shown as long ago as in the 1930's that if one common carotid artery is excluded from the circulation and the pressure in the region of its carotid sinus is lowered, a reflex increase in the systemic arterial pressure takes place; the blood flow in the contralateral common carotid artery is increased, while that in the femoral artery is reduced [323]. However, these experiments did not reveal the extent of the increase in blood flow in the brain itself as compared with that in the extracranial vessels of the head. Subsequent experiments, in which the volume velocity of the blood flow was measured in the internal carotid arteries, showed that with an increase in the systemic arterial pressure, the cerebral vessels are not involved in the generalized constrictor response of the arterial system; as a result of this, blood is redistributed from the periphery and the viscera into the central nervous system [32]. This finding was later confirmed by other work right up to the last decade. Thus, if the arterial pressure was raised through different causes (stimulation of the hypothalamus, lowering of the pressure in the region of the carotid receptors, stimulation of interoceptors of the internal organs, hypoxia, hypercapnia), the blood supply to the intestines, kidneys, liver, and skeletal muscles was reduced by a varied degree, while the blood supply to the heart and to the brain as a rule was increased [199]. Unfortunately, in most of these investigations, the methods used to record the blood flow did not give quantitative results, and they could not therefore demonstrate whether a direct relationship exists between elevation of the arterial pressure and an increase in the blood flow into the brain. The absence of active responses of the brain vessels to changes in systemic arterial pressure could also have resulted from the specific conditions of the short-term experiments under which the normal functioning of mechanisms ensuring the constancy of the cerebral circulation during changes in systemic arterial pressure was disturbed.

Improved physiological techniques, beginning with the 1950s, yielded new experimental data which indicated that, because of active responses of the brain vessels, the cerebral circulation remained more or less stable in its parameters despite considerable fluctuations in the arterial pressure. For instance, experiments on dogs showed that during a decrease in the systemic arterial pressure following bleeding, the blood supply to the head was reduced relatively less than that to other parts of the body [162]. This effect has been demonstrated

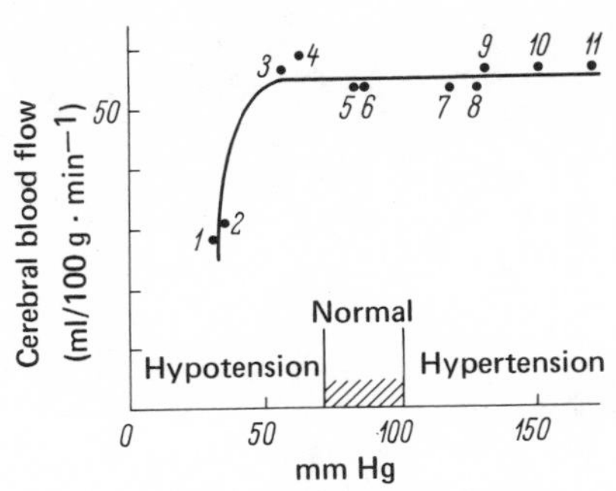

Fig. 8. Cerebral circulation in man in relation to systemic arterial pressure [170]. Mean values for 11 groups of 376 subjects (from seven papers by different authors): 1-4) hypotension of varied intensity produced by pharmacological action; 5,6) normal arterial pressure in healthy men and women; 7) hypertension produced by pharmacological action; 8) hypertensive toxemia of pregnancy; 9-11) essential hypertension.

very conclusively by Carlyle and Grayson [40] in experiments on cats when, in spite of a decrease of up to 30 mm Hg in the systemic arterial pressure the cerebral blood flow remained stable; if the pressure fell below this level the blood flow in the cerebral cortex began to decrease. Measurements of the blood flow in the cerebral cortex of monkeys by means of a thermistor showed [263] an insignificant decrease in intensity of the circulation when the systemic arterial pressure fell by 20 mm Hg, but if the systemic pressure fell to the critical level of 50-60 mm Hg the cortical blood supply started to decrease considerably and the oxygen tension in the cortex fell. Autoregulation of the cerebral circulation of this type was subsequently shown in animal experiments by many other researchers [318, 171, 114, 105, 408, 166, 34, etc.]. Quantitative measurements of the circulation in the brain of unanesthetized persions undertaken by many investigators using the Kety–Schmidt technique [143] have shown that the blood flow in the brain remains unchanged despite a considerable rise or fall of the systemic arterial pressure under different conditions. This is clearly evident in Fig. 8 [170], which generalizes the results obtained by several different investigators; impairment of the circulation in the brain begins only when the level of hypotension is considerable. All these facts indicate that, due to active responses of the blood vessels of the brain, the intensity of the cerebral circulation may remain relatively independent of the arterial pressure.

The next stage of the investigations of the cerebral circulation with which the present book is concerned is to determine which parts of the vascular system of the brain are responsible for this autoregulation. Considering the important role of the arterial system in regulating the inflow of blood into the brain (as well as in any other organ), it might be supposed that this is in fact the effector mechanism which maintains the normal cerebral circulation during changes in the systemic arterial pressure.

Role of the Major Arteries in Maintaining a Constant Inflow of Blood into the Circle of Willis

A change in the lumen of any part of a peripheral artery is reflected in its resistance, and controls both the volume velocity of blood flowing in it and also the level of the blood pressure at the periphery. Taking this into consideration, the functional behavior of the major arteries of the brain (the internal carotid and vertebral arteries) can be estimated if the pressures in them are measured simultaneously at their beginning and end, i.e., in the aorta and in the circle of Willis (or in either the basilar artery or the initial portion of the middle cerebral artery which lie close to it). By experiments of this type, many investigators have shown that pulse fluctuations in the aorta are many times greater than in the circle of Willis. This was observed originally by the use of mercury manometers [32, 296], and subsequently by means of electromanometers [363, 383, 8] and piezomanometers [286, 279, 281], which have much lower inertia. Hence it can be concluded that the pulse fluctuations are largely damped out along the course of the major arteries supplying blood to the brain. It was postulated originally [148] that this takes place because of the existence of curvatures* in the internal carotid and vertebral arteries. However, we now know that the same phenomenon takes place in animals which have no curvatures (in rabbits, for example). This indicates an active role of the arterial walls in the processes involved in damping the pulse fluctuations of systemic arterial pressure, although it does not rule out entirely the role of curvatures in these arteries in animals which possess them.

*The present author decided not to use the widely accepted term "siphon," since the curvature of the internal carotid artery resembles a siphon only in its shape, not in its fluid mechanics.

Results indicating that relatively slow fluctuations of systemic arterial pressure, such as respiratory waves and third-order waves of Traube–Hering, undergo active elimination in the system of the major arteries of the brain have also been obtained in experiments giving indirect evidence of the functional state of the major arteries of the brain, namely the velocity of spread of the pulse wave from the aorta to the circle of Willis: with each inspiration and each rise of arterial pressure, it increased, indicating an increase in the "tone" of the internal carotid and vertebral arteries, i.e., indicating their constriction. A similar process affects the time of the third-order waves, which are of much greater amplitude [283].

This damping of the various types of fluctuations of systemic arterial pressure results in a relatively constant level of pressure in the brain vessels. This may be of considerable physiological importance, because the brain is situated inside the rigid cranium, and is surrounded by cerebrospinal fluid, so that any fluctuations of intravascular pressure must exert a mechanical effect on tissue elements of the brain. However, under normal conditions this does not take place, since the fluctuations of pressure in the cerebral arteries are reduced to a minimum, as a result of their damping in the system of the internal carotid and vertebral arteries.

Comparatively longer changes in the lumen and resistance of the major arteries of the brain can naturally lead to changes in the blood pressure in the circle of Willis which are relatively independent of the level of systemic arterial pressure. The fact that the levels of the systemic arterial pressure and the pressure in the circle of Willis do not run parallel to each other was observed as long ago as the last century [118]; this indicated that the pressure drop along the major arteries of the brain may differ. In later experiments [22], during spontaneous fluctuations in the level of the systemic arterial pressure, the blood pressure in the circle of Willis changed in the opposite direction every time, an increase in its pressure being combined with increased outflow of blood from the jugular vein; the pressure gradient along the major arteries of the brain varied in these experiments from 24 to 58 mm Hg, indicating corresponding changes of resistance along these vessels. No parallel likewise was found between the pressure levels in human subjects when measured simultaneously in the brachial (systemic arterial pressure) and pial arteries [179].

Experimental results obtaining during the last 15 years indicate that the resistance in the major arteries of the brain, (judged from the pressure gradient in them) can vary with the level of the systemic arterial pressure, and that the direction of these changes is perfectly regular. During stimulation of the carotid sinus, for instance, the systemic pressure falls more severely than the pressure in the circle of Willis [407]. Conversely, in the case of a pressor response of the systemic arterial pressure, e.g., to stimulation of the carotid sinus or mechanoreceptors of the spleen [309] or of the proprioceptors of striated muscles [54], the increase in systemic arterial pressure is always greater than the increase in pressure in the circle of Willis. The same phenomenon was observed when the systemic arterial pressure and the pressure in the basilar artery were measured simultaneously; after injection of adrenalin the pressure in the first increased more than in the second [363]. All these results may indicate that elevation of the systemic arterial pressure is accompanied by an increase of resistance in the major arteries of the brain. This increase evidently results from constriction of these arteries, more especially because the pial arteries, which lie peripherally to the circle of Willis, also are constricted under these conditions (see pp. 20 and 21), and cannot be responsible for the reduction in blood pressure in the circle of Willis.

Further experiments showed that such responses of the internal carotid and vertebral arteries frequently do not develop immediately. If the level of the systemic arterial pressure was raised repeatedly at intervals of a few minutes (through intravenous injections of equal doses of adrenalin), initially the pressure in the circle of Willis also rose (although to a lesser degree), but the third and fourth times it remained unchanged (Fig. 9) [211]. Subsequent control tests showed that after repeated injections of adrenalin directly into the isolated internal carotid artery *in situ* the resistance in it (the perfusion pressure in this artery was measured) changes almost equally every time; consequently, the gradually developing constrictor response of the major arteries to the brain in the above experiments was due, not to the direct action of adrenalin on the walls of these arteries, but to the repeated elevation of the systemic arterial pressure.

Since the pressure gradient along the major arteries of the brain is an indirect index of the resistance in these arteries, and because of the great difficulty presented by the measurement of this resistance in physiological experiments, a mathematical model has now been developed to enable it to

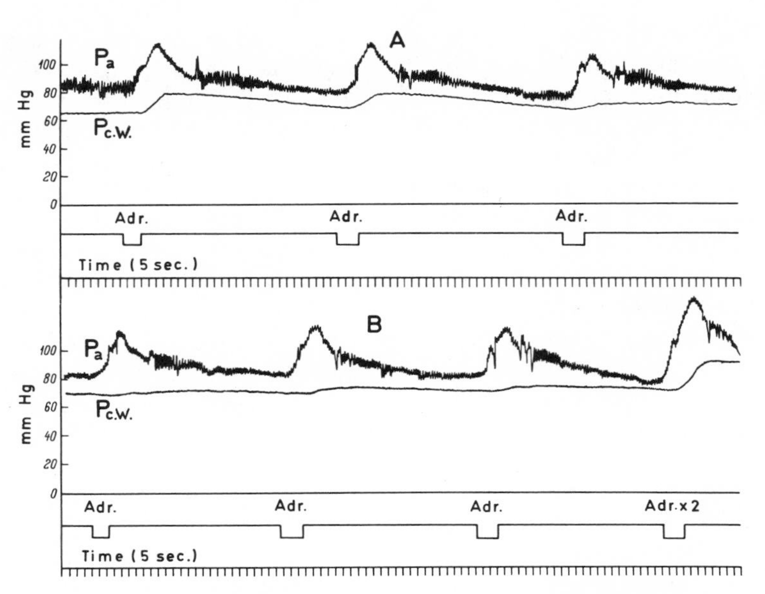

Fig. 9. Increase in resistance in major arteries of the rabbit's brain after repeated elevation of the systemic arterial pressure through intravenous injection of adrenalin (1×10^{-4}) in a volume of 0.1 ml; at the seventh injection the dose was doubled [211]. Explanation in text. P_a, arterial pressure in aorta; $P_{c.W.}$, pressure in circle of Willis. B, direct continuation of trace A.

be calculated (see p. 11). If the systemic arterial pressure fell slightly, the pressure in the circle of Willis either remained unchanged or changed insignificantly. Calculation of the resistance in the major arteries of the brain from these pressures and the venous pressure in the brain sinuses showed that it was lowered, whereas the resistance in the smaller arteries located peripherally to the circle of Willis was unchanged (Fig. 10). To raise the systemic arterial pressure, the experiments were carried out as follows: the external carotid artery and all anastomoses of the internal carotid artery with the extracerebral vessels (see p. 8) were ligated in dogs and blood was then injected into this internal carotid artery (the innervation of the carotid sinus was carefully preserved) by means of a pump so that the level of the input pressure could be altered. These experiments showed that, when the input pressure was raised, the resistance in the internal carotid artery was increased and the pressure in the circle of Willis thus remained almost unchanged. The resistance in the arteries located peripherally to the circle of Willis also remained unchanged (Fig. 11). The results of these experiments thus provide direct proof that autoregulation of the cerebral circulation can be carried out by those major arteries of the brain one of whose functions it is to ensure a constant inflow of blood into the circle of Willis, despite considerable fluctuations in the systemic arterial pressure.

Functional Behavior of the Pial, Precortical, and Cortical Arteries during Changes of the Systemic Arterial Pressure

As early as the 1930's it was observed in experiments on cats that if the systemic arterial pressure falls to 70 mm Hg (as a result of stimulation of the vagus nerve), the pial arteries, which were investigated directly under the microscope, begin to dilate [79]. This effect occurred when the arterial pressure fell for various reasons: the lower the pressure, the more the pial arteries dilated [75]. In another investigation [314] the pial arteries responded distinctly to lowering of the systemic arterial pressure (resulting from administration of the ganglion-blocking drug hexamethonium) by 25 mm Hg from its initial level; if the pressure fell by less than 15 mm, no effect was observed. Dilatation of the pial arteries has been observed also during systemic arterial hypotension caused by bleeding [3, 71].

During elevation of the systemic arterial pressure, the opposite response of the pial arteries has been observed: they constrict. In experiments on cats [76] constriction of the pial arteries took

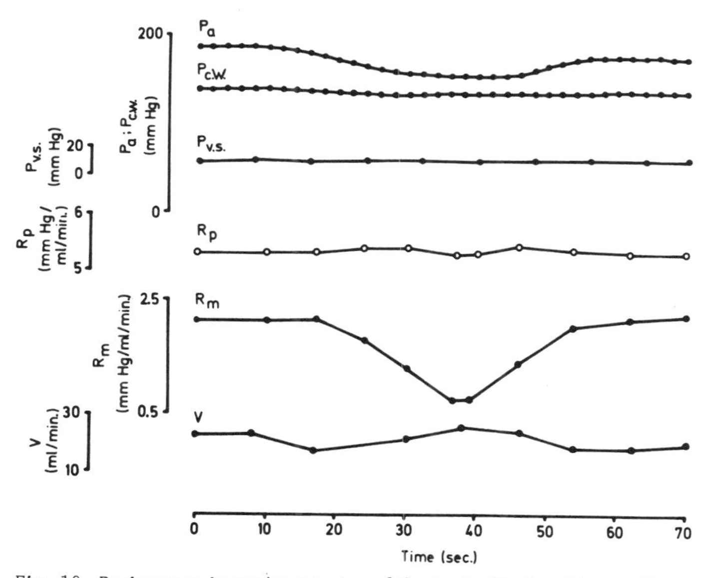

Fig. 10. Resistances in major arteries of the brain (R_m) and in small arteries peripherally to circle of Willis (R_p) calculated by the use of a mathematical model from pressures recorded in physiological experiments on dog in aorta (P_a) and circle of Willis (P_{cW}) and in venous sinuses of brain (P_{vs}) during a spontaneous decrease in systemic arterial pressure (experiments performed by the author in conjuction with N. P. Mitagvariya and L. G. Ormotsadze).

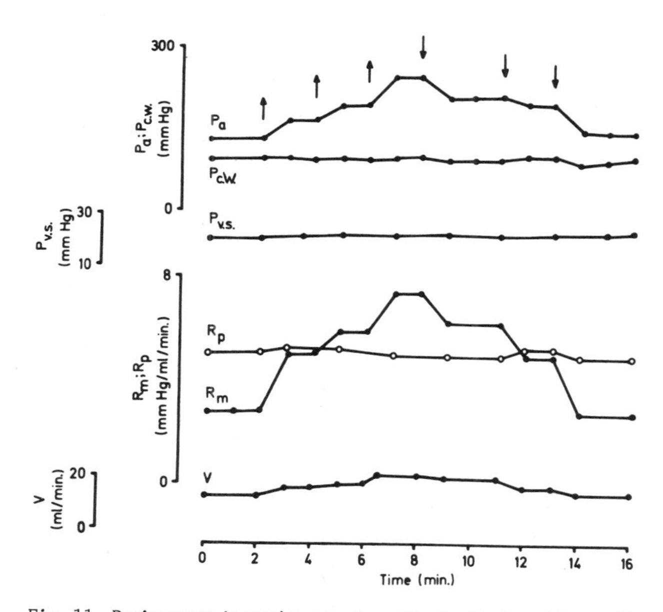

Fig. 11. Resistances in major arteries of brain (R_m) and in small arteries peripherally to circle of Willis (R_p) calculated, by means of a mathematical model, from perfusion pressure in internal carotid artery isolated in situ (P_a), pressure in circle of Willis (P_{cW}), and pressure in venous sinuses of brain (P_{vs}) recorded in experiments on a dog during artificial change in perfusion pressure resulting from changes in output of pump (indicated by arrows). Volume velocity of blood flow calculated from results obtained [248].

place when the systemic arterial pressure rose by more than 20% of its initial level, and this constriction was particularly clear if the initial pressure was low. In response to a very considerable increase in arterial pressure [39], for example to 200 mm Hg in rats (after extirpation of one kidney and compression of the opposite renal artery), constriction of the pial arteries resembled spasm, cortical function was disturbed, and local edema and even necrosis of the brain tissue developed. The constrictor response of the pial arteries is evidently the result of an increase of intravascular pressure in the head. Evidence in favor of this is given by experiments (on cats and dogs) in which constriction of the vessels took place not only in response to an increase in aortic pressure (application of a screw clamp to descending aorta), but also during elevation of pressure in the blood vessels of the head only (injection of blood into the carotid artery); under these circumstances constriction of the pial arteries (with a diameter of 40-250 μ) reached 50% of their initial diameter [264].

The relationship between the amplitude of responses of the pial arteries and the caliber of the vessels, as well as the time of appearance of these responses have recently been studied in experiments on rabbits [253]. When the systemic arterial pres-

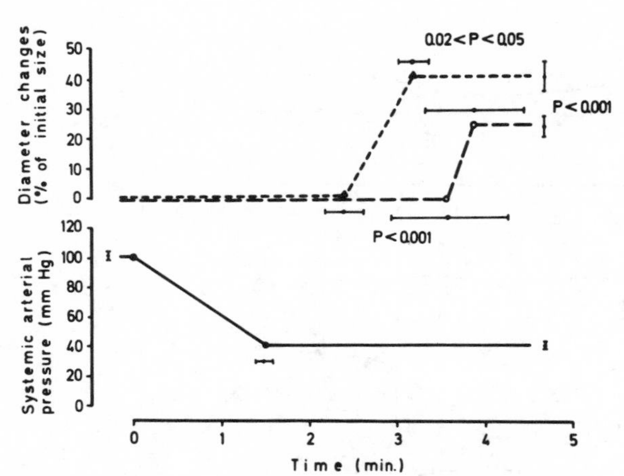

Fig. 12. Degree and time of dilatation of pial arteries less than 100 μ (dotted line) and more than 100 μ (broken line) in caliber during stepwise decrease in systemic arterial pressure in a rabbit. Arithmetic mean values and confidence limits shown [253].

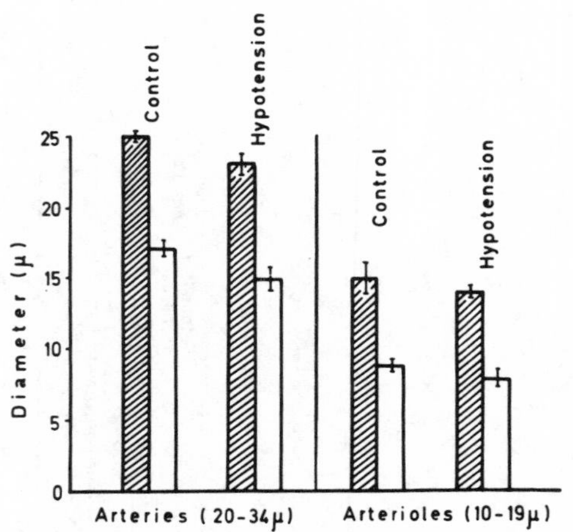

Fig. 13. External diameter (shaded columns) and diameter of lumen (unshaded columns) of small arteries and arterioles in rabbit cortex in control experiments (systemic arterial pressure about 100 mm Hg) and in arterial hypotension (about 40 mm Hg). Arithmetic mean values and confidence limits shown [253].

sure was lowered on the average from 101 to 41 mm Hg, the small pial arteries (less than 100 μ in caliber) did not start to dilate until after 142 ± 14 sec, and the large arteries (more than 100 μ in caliber) until later still, after 214 ± 40 sec ($P < 0.001$). The small pial arteries also stopped dilating as a rule earlier than the large arteries, after 182 ± 10 and 230 ± 34 sec respectively. The degree of dilatation of the pial arteries of different caliber also differed: whereas the small pial arteries dilated by 40 ± 5%, the large arteries dilated by 24 ± 4% of their initial value ($P < 0.001$; Fig. 12).

Measurement of the diameter of the cortical arteries and arterioles after intravital fixation of the vessels showed [253] that not only was their width during hypotension not greater than in the control, but it was actually slightly less (Fig. 13), i.e., unlike the pial arteries, these cortical arteries do not participate in autoregulatory dilatation of the cerebral vessels.

Responses of the precortical arteries (intermediate portions between the pial and cortical arteries) in rabbits with hypertension and hypotension have also recently been investigated [236]. Along the length of the precortical arteries there was an active portion the lumen of which was considerably constricted during an increase in the systemic arterial pressure by 50-70 mm Hg as the result of intravenous infusion of noradrenalin (Fig. 14). In hypotension due to withdrawal of blood into the reservoir of the compensator, on the other hand, when the systemic arterial pressure was reduced on the average to 35 mm Hg, no statistically significant changes in diameter of the precortical arteries compared with the control were found (Fig. 14). In hypertension, precortical arteries more than 25 μ in caliber were constricted to a greater degree than the smaller arteries. In their constricted portions, the smooth-muscle cells were contracted, for their nuclei were much shorter than in the control. Where the precortical arteries were constricted, their lumen was on the average 35% smaller than that of the corresponding radial arteries entering the cortex (in the control they were always larger, on the average by 32%).

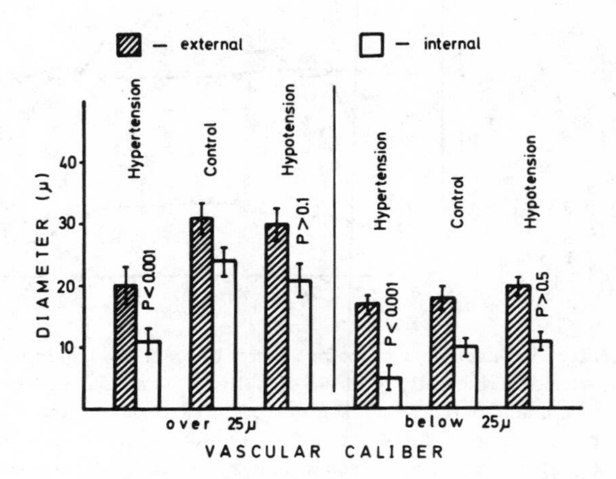

Fig. 14. Functional behavior of large and small precortical arteries of rabbits with arterial hypertension and hypotension. Arithmetic mean values and confidence limits shown [236].

Hence, as the systemic arterial pressure is lowered, dilatation of the pial arteries takes place regularly, but after such a long delay that this vasodilatation can hardly be regarded as a direct manifestation of autoregulation, i.e., the stimulus evoking responses of the pial arteries cannot be the change in intravascular pressure. In some recent experiments [253] it always came on after the inflow of blood into the cortex had been reduced, and the value of pO_2 in the cortex had fallen. These results suggest that dilatation of the pial arteries is in all probability the response of these vessels to an insufficient inflow of blood into the cortex. In other words, when the systemic arterial pressure falls, dilatation of the pial arteries is apparently a reserve autoregulatory mechanism which begins to function if the major arteries can no longer ensure a constant intracranial inflow of blood, as the result either of excessively large changes in systemic arterial pressure or of disturbances of the function of this vascular mechanism. So far as the increases in systemic arterial pressure are concerned, the available experimental data are not yet sufficient to explain the role of the pial and smaller vessels of the brain in this regulation.

Functional Insufficiency of Vascular Mechanisms during Changes in Systemic Arterial Pressure

There is a critical level, which is not always the same, of the systemic arterial pressure below which the cerebral blood flow begins to decrease. It was shown that when the systemic arterial pressure fell in man to between 29 and 89 mm Hg, the blood supply to the brain remained unchanged [72]. The existence of such a critical level of arterial pressure, differing from one subject to another, indicates that the vascular mechanisms of the brain compensating these changes in its perfusion pressure do not function identically in different people. The possibility is not ruled out that in the course of each person's or animal's life this critical level of arterial pressure may change, first, with the onset of pathological changes in the walls of the cerebral vessels (arteriosclerosis) and second, through changes in the functional state of the physiological mechanisms of compensation. Naturally this regulatory mechanism, operating through the major arteries of the brain, has limited possibilities. If fluctuations of the systemic arterial pressure are relatively great, they cannot be abolished within the extent of these arteries and they appear in the circle of Willis (usually in a more or less attenuated form). In these cases the intravascular pressure also changes in the smaller arteries and the blood supply to the cerebral tissue becomes altered; this, in turn, may lead to active changes in the diameter of the lumen of the pial and precortical arteries.

The normal functional behavior of the mechanisms of autoregulation of the cerebral circulation with the participation of the major arteries of the brain (and, possibly, of the pial arteries) can easily be disturbed. This was shown in experiments in which animals were anesthetized or had received ganglion-blocking drugs [289], or had undergone a severe surgical operation such as isolation of an area of the cerebral cortex [361] or ligation of relatively inaccessible vessels in the region of the skull [337]. Further investigations showed that the autoregulation of the cerebral circulation can easily be abolished after brain trauma [325], or after cerebral ischemia [402, 172]. It was abolished also in hypercapnia [321, 171, 102, 106, 157] and hypoxia [100, 77, 82], evidently, at least partly, because of the considerable dilatation of the cerebral vessels under these conditions.

Though the blood supply to the brain, when measured in hypertensive subjects, as a rule is not increased [170, 142, 52], the compensatory mechanisms of the major arteries of the brain are sometimes slow in warming up (Fig. 9), and this explains why sudden increases in arterial pressure in hypertensive subjects [e.g., 384], when the blood pressure must also increase in the vessels of the brain, are so dangerous, for if changes are also present in the vessel walls hemorrhages and other cerebrovascular disturbances may appear. The various cerebral manifestations of arterial hypertension may thus represent the result of disturbances of compansation of the raised systemic arterial pressure by the major and other arteries of the brain.

CHAPTER III

INTRACRANIAL CIRCULATORY DISORDERS

A vital step in the study of differences between the functions of different parts of the cerebrovascular system is the investigation of their behavior under different conditions and, in particular in cerebrovascular disturbances which are either unaccompanied or accompanied by a marked deficiency in the blood supply to the brain tissues. The disorders in which there is no primary or marked deficiency of blood supply to the brain tissue include, for example, traumatic cerebral edema and the transient intracranial venous stagnation following occlusion of the jugular veins in the neck. A deficiency in blood supply is also found in the presence of severe venous stasis during occlusion of the cranial vena cava, in general asphyxia through occlusion of the trachea, and in postischemic states of the brain. A deficiency in the blood supply arises in circumscribed areas of the cerebral cortex at times of a sharp increase in its activity as the result, for example, of application of strychnine, and when ischemic foci arise in the cortex through occlusion of the pial arteries. The functional behavior of the vascular mechanisms of the brain has also been studied under conditions when a collateral circulation becomes necessary after occlusion of the cerebral arteries. Finally, the study of responses of the cerebral vessels during terminal states as death approaches is of great interest from this point of view.

Occlusion of Jugular Veins (Mild and Transient Stagnation of Venous Blood)

Transient stagnation of blood with an insignificant increase in blood pressure in the venous system of the brain may arise after simultaneous occlusion of all the jugular veins in the animal's neck. By recording several parameters of the cerebral circulation, the functional behavior of the blood vessels and changes in circulation of the blood into the brain were studied under these conditions in 42 rabbits [207, 209]. The level of the systemic arterial pressure remained unchanged, but measurements of the retrograde outflow of blood from the circle of Willis through one of the internal carotid arteries showed it to be considerably reduced (Fig. 15); the same result was found after ligation of the animal's second carotid artery. Since the largest veins of the brain were ligated, and this was bound to interfere with drainage of blood into the extracranial venous system, the observed effect could only depend on a decrease in the inflow of blood into the circle of Willis along the major arteries of the brain: the contralateral internal carotid artery and the two vertebral arteries. This conclusion was also supported by the decrease in blood pressure in the pial arteries, recorded by estimation of the external pressure necessary to compress the vessels (Fig. 16). Serial photomicrography of the pial arteries, followed by their measurement on the photographic film showed that their diameter was regularly reduced, on the average by 18 ± 1.7% of its initial value (Fig. 17). This indicates that under these conditions constriction affects both the major arteries of the brain and the pial arteries. As a result of this vasoconstriction, some reduction in the blood flow into the brain was inevitable. In fact, investigation of the diameter of the pial veins by serial photomicrography showed transient dilatation followed frequently by constriction. The char-

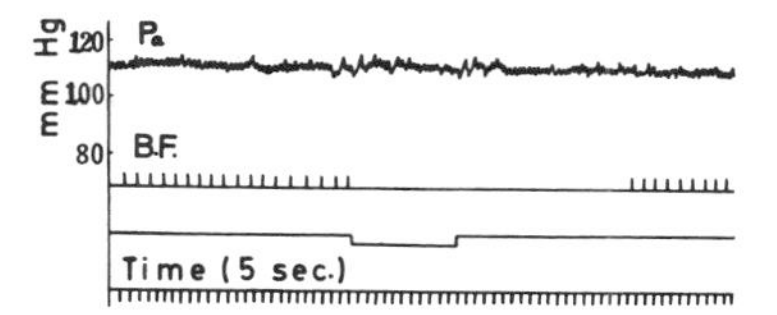

Fig. 15. Reduction in inflow of blood into circle of Willis along major arteries of the brain following simultaneous occlusion of jugular veins in the neck of a rabbit [209]. Explanation in text. P_a, systemic arterial pressure; B.F., recording of drops of blood escaping along right internal carotid artery from circle of Willis.

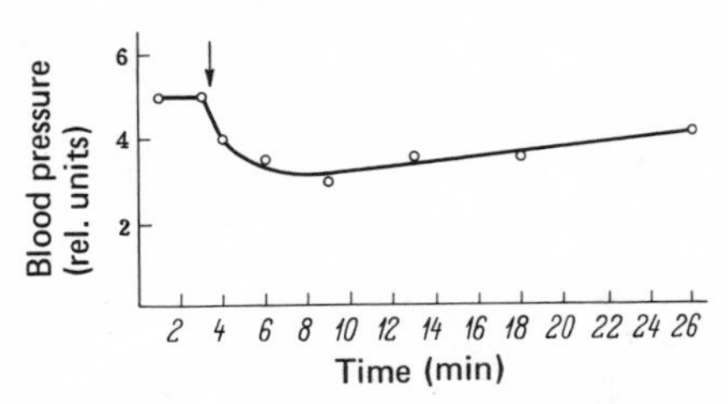

Fig. 16. Decrease in blood pressure in pial arteries after simultaneous occlusion of external jugular veins in a rabbit (time of occlusion marked by an arrow). Method of indirect pressure measurement described in [209].

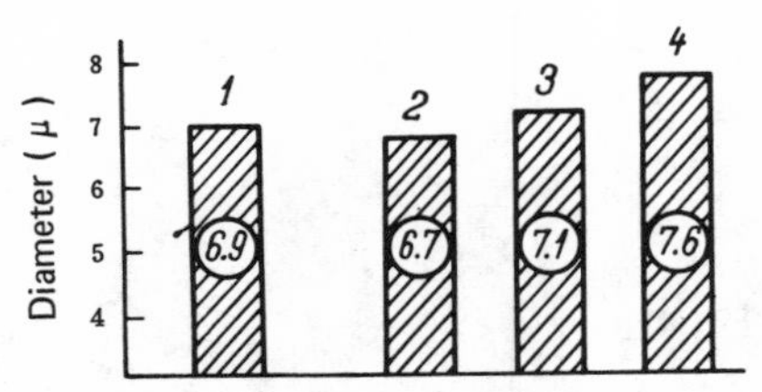

Fig. 18. Diameter of capillaries (mean value) in parietal cortex of rabbits under different conditions [209]. Explanation in text. 1) after occlusion of jugular veins; 2) in control experiments; 3) during inhalation of gas mixture with increased CO_2 concentration; 4) in aseptic inflammation of the pia mater.

acteristic picture of their changes is shown in Fig. 17: for the first minute after ligation of the jugular veins the pial veins were dilated, but later (after 4.5 min) they were constricted to their original diameter, after which they became narrower than initially. Investigation of the capillaries in the intravitally fixed parietal cortex showed (Fig. 18) that, after ligation of the jugular veins, their diameter was a little larger than in the control ($0.05 > P > 0.02$); it was slightly smaller than during inhalation of a gas mixture containing 10% CO_2 ($0.2 > P > 0.1$), and much smaller than in the presence of aseptic inflammation of the pia mater ($P < 0.001$). Direct measurements of the blood pressure with a water manometer in the sagittal venous sinus and in the large veins of the brain surface also systematically revealed (starting from 2-3 min) a decrease, followed by a return to its initial value. The decrease in venous pressure in the brain sinuses was slight, and did not exceed 1-2 mm Hg. But it undoubtedly indicated not only the absence of venous stagnation in the brain, but also a decrease in the inflow of blood into the brain, for even the most perfect collateral drainage from the skull could not have lowered the pressure in the cerebral veins (all the jugular veins having been ligated). The intensity of outflow of blood from the catheter tied into the sagittal sinus fell appreciably in most (82%) experiments after 2-3 min, and sometimes stopped completely for a time, although the systemic arterial pressure remained unchanged* (Fig. 19). This effect gave direct evidence of a reduction in the in-

* The initial increase in outflow of venous blood (in the period of transient blood stagnation) was not always detected in these experiments, probably because the method used possessed relatively high inertia.

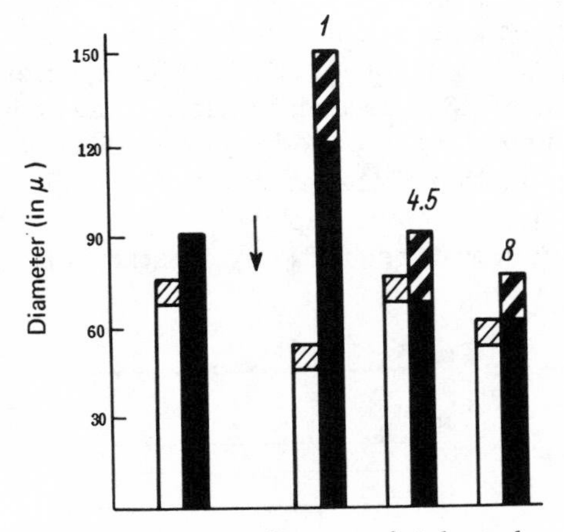

Fig. 17. Changes in diameter of pial vessels after simultaneous occlusion of external jugular veins in rabbits [209]. Unshaded columns represent artery, black columns vein; shaded parts of columns give limits of periodic fluctuations in diameter of vessels. Numbers above columns show time after occlusion of jugular veins (in min); arrow indicates occlusion.

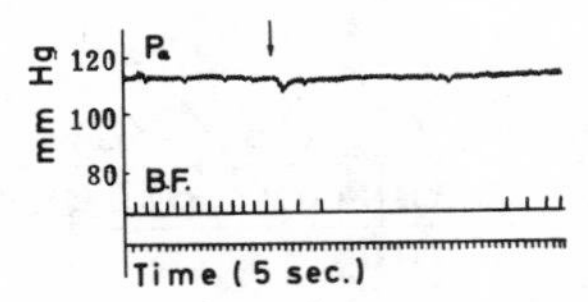

Fig. 19. Intensity of outflow of blood from sagittal sinus after simultaneous occlusion of external jugular veins in a rabbit [209]. Explanation in text. P_a, systemic arterial pressure; B.F., recording of drops of blood escaping from sinus. Arrow indicates time of occlusion.

flow of blood into the brain immediately after occlusion of the jugular veins.

Transient stagnation of blood developing in the venous system of the brain following simultaneous occlusion of the external and internal jugular vein in an animal's neck thus produces constriction both of the system of major arteries and of the pial arteries. As a result, the inflow of blood into the brain is to some extent reduced, and this cannot but reduce the stagnation of venous blood in the brain. It can therefore be supposed that the constrictor response of the brain arteries described above is compensatory, for if blood continued to enter the brain vessels, the outflow from which was reduced, under its usual high pressure, marked signs of stagnation of blood would develop in all the blood vessels of the brain. Such a disturbance of the circulation would be particularly dangerous for the brain, not only because of the high sensitivity of its tissue to disturbances of blood supply, but also because it is situated inside the rigid box of the skull, and therefore the pressure around its tissue elements would be significantly increased.

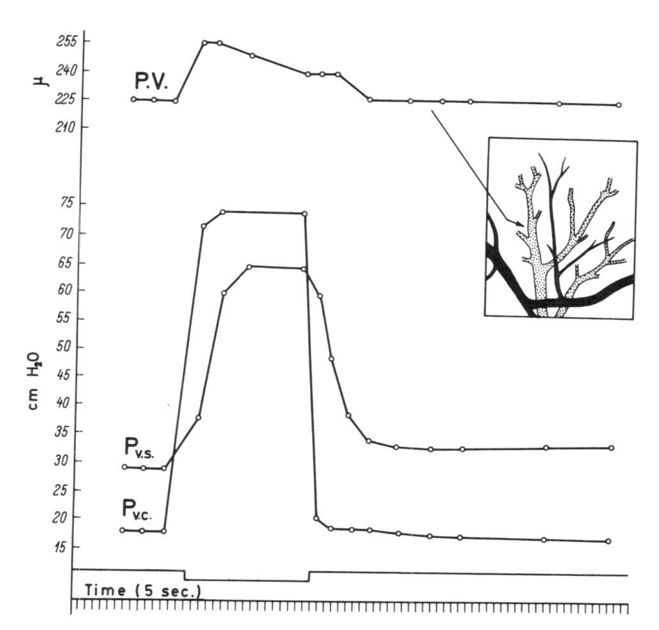

Fig. 20. Dynamics of the venous pressures and active constriction of a dilated pial vein during occlusion of the cranial vena cava in a dog [232]. P.V., diameter of pial vein (indicated in the diagram on the right); $P_{v.s.}$, venous pressure in transverse sinus; $P_{v.c.}$, pressure in cranial vena cava.

Severe Stagnation of Blood in the Cerebral Vessels Resulting from Occlusion of the Cranial (Superior) Vena Cava

Although because of the well developed compensatory mechanisms (the numerous anastomoses in the venous system of the brain and, in particular, responses of the major arteries of the brain and the pial arteries), blood stagnation cannot be produced in the brain by occlusion even of most of the larger venous trunks in the animal's neck, considerable stagnation of blood in the cerebral vessels does occur, however, after occlusion of the cranial vena cava in dogs [232]. To reduce the likelihood of a collateral venous drainage, the azygos vein was first ligated, since in experiments on dogs, after occlusion of the cranial vena cava the blood flow in the cortex, measured by the radioactive krypton clearance method, was not significantly changed if the azygos vein was not ligated; the blood flow was reduced only after ligation of that vein [134]. In the authors' experiments on dogs [232], immediately after occlusion of the cranial vena cava the blood pressure in the brain sinuses rose from 20 ± 0.8 to 50 ± 1.3 cm water, i.e., by 2.5 times ($P < 0.001$), and remained at this level (sometimes falling gradually) throughout the period of occlusion of the vena cava (Fig. 20). As a result, the pressure gradient in the cerebral vessels was reduced: the difference between the pressure in the circle of Willis and the venous sinuses of the brain was then 26 ± 5.4 mm Hg, compared with 57 ± 7 mm Hg before occlusion of the vena cava, i.e., it was reduced by more than half ($P < 0.001$). This naturally caused a marked decrease in the velocity of the blood flow in the arteries and veins on the brain surface, indicating a corresponding slowing of the circulation of blood also in the cortical capillaries.

The primary slowing of the blood flow which must have occurred in the major arteries of the brain prevented the functional state of these arteries from being judged by the pressure gradient in them. However, immediately after restoration of the patency of the cranial vena cava and the elimination of intracranial blood stagnation, it became evident that the pressure difference between the aorta and circle of Willis was increased in every case, from 26 ± 0.3 to 35 ± 0.5 mm Hg, i.e., by 36% of the initial value ($P < 0.001$) (Fig. 21). This therefore suggested that when considerable blood stagnation exists in the cerebrovascular system and is probably accompanied by the development of edema (as shown by an increase in brain volume demonstrable after removal of the occlusion of the cranial vena cava), the system of major arteries of the brain apparently undergoes constriction in the

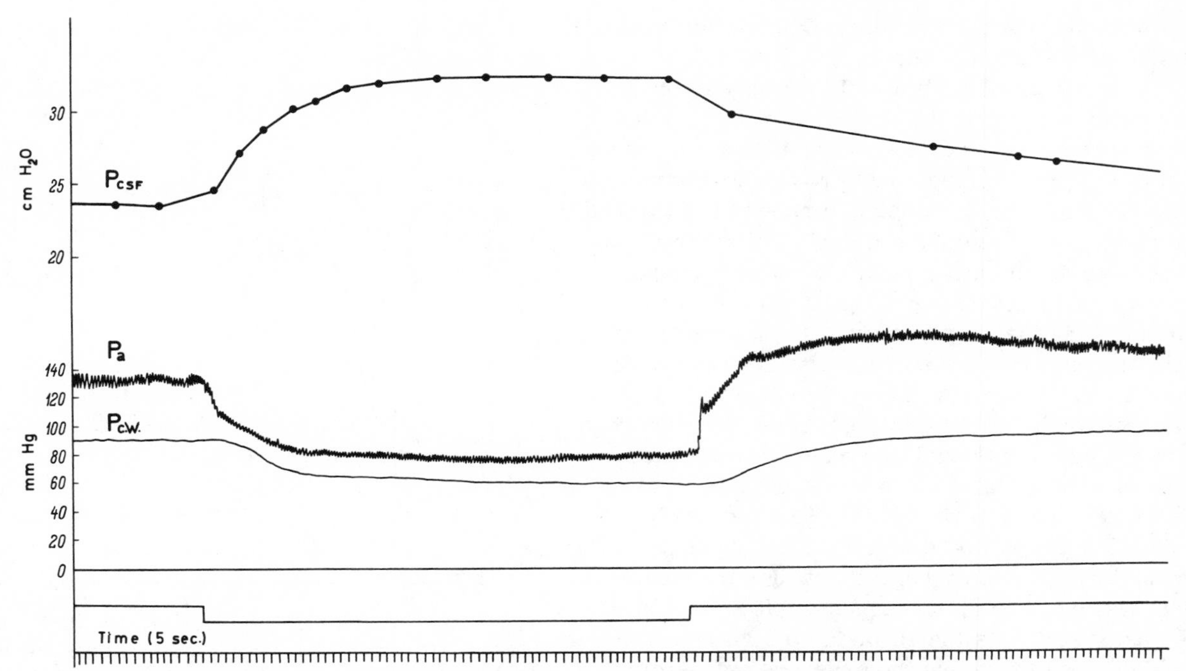

Fig. 21. Arterial pressure and pressure gradient in major arteries of the brain during and after occlusion of cranial (superior) vena cava in a dog [232]. P_{csf}, intracranial pressure; P_a, systemic arterial pressure; $P_{c.W.}$, pressure in circle of Willis. Marker shows time of occlusion of cranial vena cava.

same way as in the presence of mild stagnation in the brain. It is only very recently that the resistance in the major arteries of the brain during occlusion of the cranial vena cava could be calculated with the aid of a mathematical model from pressures recorded in the aorta, circle of Willis, and venous sinuses of the brain. It will be clear from Fig. 22 that the resistance in the major arteries of the brain was increased under these circumstances (just as it was when mild venous stagnation followed occlusion of the jugular veins), and the resistance peripherally to the circle of Willis, after an initial transient increase, then began to fall progressively, presumably through gradual dilatation of the pial arteries. The blood flow into the brain, calculated by means of the same mathematical model, was reduced under these conditions.

So far as functional behavior of the pial arteries during occlusion of the cranial vena cava is concerned (when the blood flow in the cerebral capillaries is considerably slowed and the blood supply to the brain must be certainly deficient, as a rule they were dilated [232]. Changes in the diameter of pial arteries of different caliber before and after occlusion of the vena cava in dogs showed the char-

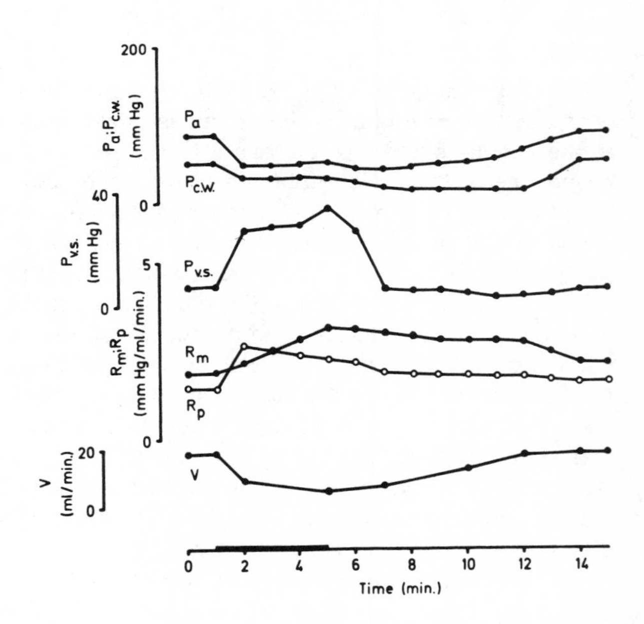

Fig. 22. Resistance in major arteries of brain (R_m) and in small arteries peripherally to circle of Willis (R_p) calculated with the aid of a mathematical model from pressures recorded in physiological experiments in aorta (P_a), in circle of Willis (P_{cW}), and in venous sinuses of brain (P_{vs}) during occlusion of cranial vena cava in a dog. Volume velocity of blood flow calculated from results obtained [248].

acteristic features distinguishing the responses of larger and smaller arteries. The wider arteries (over 225 μ in diameter) were slightly constricted at the beginning of occlusion, but by not more than 10% of their initial diameter, and later they began to dilate; during repeated occlusions this initial constriction gradually became weaker and, finally, it disappeared altogether and only dilatation of the pial arteries was observed. The smaller the diameter of these vessels, the more marked their dilatation. Measurement of the diameter of many of these vessels showed that arteries with an initial diameter of 80-120 μ dilated by 20-60%, and those with a diameter of 30-45 μ dilated by 85-175% of their diameter. Considering that this dilatation of the pial arteries must reduce the resistance to the blood flow and hence decrease the deficiency of blood supply to the corresponding parts of the brain, it can be concluded that the smaller the diameter of the pial arteries, the more evident their nutritive role in the regulation of an adequate blood supply to the brain tissue.

Thus, in contrast to mild stagnation of blood, of short duration, in the venous system of the brain (produced by occlusion of the jugular veins in the neck), during severe stagnation affecting the whole vascular system of the brain, when the blood flow in its capillaries is considerably slowed, causing a deficiency of the blood supply to its tissues (occlusion of the cranial vena cava), the pial arteries are not constricted but, on the contrary, they become dilated, and the smaller the caliber of the vessels, the more marked this dilatation. So far as the system of major arteries of the brain is concerned, in both cases it behaves simularly: these arteries constrict and increase the resistance to the blood flow along the path to the circle of Willis.

The systemic arterial pressure also takes part in the compensation of cerebrovascular disturbances after occlusion of the cranial (superior) vena cava, when considerable stagnation of blood develops in the cerebral vessels. In experiments on dogs the arterial pressure fell at once and remained at about the same level throughout the period of occlusion, sometimes rising or falling gradually (Fig. 20). It fell on the average from 106 ± 5 to 74 ± 5 mm Hg, and this led to a decrease in the blood pressure in the circle of Willis on the average from 69 ± 8.6 to 60 ± 7.5 mm Hg ($P < 0.001$) [232]. This must have led to a relative decrease in the intracapillary pressure and, consequently, it must have limited the development of cerebral edema. Lowering of the arterial pressure after occlusion of the superior vena cava has also been observed in man during surgical operations [98], and the absence of this compensatory reaction considerably aggravated the patient's condition and frequently led to his death.

Traumatic Cerebral Edema

In traumatic cerebral edema, the circulation in the brain is disturbed but there is no primary and well-marked deficiency of its blood supply. The main changes are found in the blood–brain barrier, whose permeability is increased, so that water passes from the blood into the brain tissues in excess, together with the salts dissolved in it, colloidal particles, and even erythrocytes. An increase in permeability of the walls of the blood vessels of the brain in cerebral edema arising from various causes has been demonstrated by several different methods. If trypan blue [316, 38], radioactive isotopes [9, 138, 57, 20], or fluorescent substances [146, 403] are injected into the blood stream they begin to pass through the barrier of the vessel walls into the brain tissues, which does not happen under normal circumstances. Meanwhile, if these substances are injected directly into the brain, they are retained there and are removed from it much more slowly [7].

The next problem to consider is how the different parts of the cerebrovascular system behave during the development of traumatic edema and what changes takes place in the cerebral circulation under these conditions. This problem has been studied to some extent in adult rabbits, but chiefly in dogs [227, 228, 229]. Cerebral edema was produced in some experiments by standard mechanical injury to the brain surface (cortex and immediate subcortex), and in others by electrical coagulation of an area of brain tissue (measuring 5-8 mm in diameter) in the region of the mesencephalon and diencephalon. During the period of 1-4 h after injuries of this type, generalized cerebral edema developed. Its existence was demonstrated both by local macroscopic changes and by the results of subsequent histological examinations of the brain tissue. During the time between injury of the brain and the appearance of appreciable edema, two consecutive responses of the cerebral arterial system were observed: the first in the period preceding the appearance of marked edema, i.e., in the period of "pre-edema," and the second after the appearance of edema.

During the period of pre-edema, the pressure difference between the aorta and circle of Willis (with a comparable level of the systemic arterial pressure) in all cases became smaller (Fig. 23B). In experiments on dogs this difference was reduced

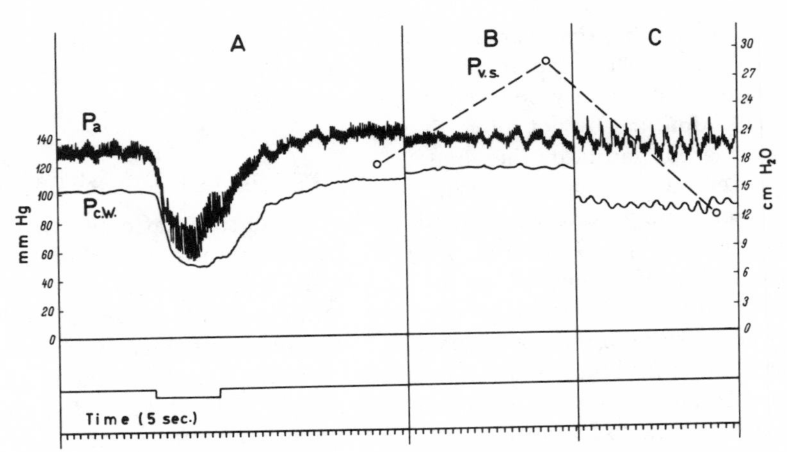

Fig. 23. Changes of pressure gradient in major arteries of the brain and venous pressure in the transverse sinus during development of traumatic cerebral edema in dogs [227, 228]. P_a, blood pressure in aorta; $P_{c.W.}$, pressure in circle of Willis (scale of the left); $P_{v.s.}$, venous pressure in sagittal sinus (scale on the right). The marker shows the period of brain trauma. A) In period of injury in region of mesencephalon and diencephalon; B) in state of pre-edema (1 h 45 min after trauma); C) after development of edema (3 h 45 min after trauma).

from 35 ± 2.5 mm Hg to 21 ± 2.4 mm Hg, i.e., on the average by 40% ($P > 0.001$). Thus, it could be concluded that cerebral edema was preceded by a decrease in resistance along the course of the major arteries of the brain, evidently as a result of their dilatation. Meanwhile, the diameter of the pial arteries (the same vessels were measured) also increased from 129 ± 11.4 to 148 ± 22.8 μ, i.e., on the average by 15% of its initial value ($0.01 > P > 0.001$). Consequently, in the state of pre-edema, the arterial system of the brain was dilated. Simultaneously, the pressure in the venous sinuses of the brain was raised (Fig. 23B).

After the development of edema, the functional state of the internal carotid and vertebral arteries apparently changed in the opposite direction. Constriction of these arteries was demonstrated by an increase in the pressure difference between the aorta and circle of Willis (Fig. 23C). This difference increased on the average from 35 ± 2.5 to 47 ± 3.2 mm Hg, i.e., by 34% of the initial value observed before trauma ($P < 0.001$). The pial arteries also constricted after the development of edema (the diameter of the same blood vessels was measured), on the average from 129 ± 11.4 to 105 ± 19.3 μ, i.e., by 19% of their initial diameter ($0.02 > P > 0.01$). The constriction of the pial arteries during the period cannot be the result of external compression, because it is also observed when the skull is trephined and the dura opened, when the pressure in the medium surrounding these arteries could not have increased during the experiment.

In general, the faster the edema developed, the more rapidly dilatation and constriction of the arteries followed each other. If a burr-hole was simply drilled in the skull (without mechanical injury to the brain), edema developed comparatively slowly and the dilatation of the pial arteries preceding it continued for along time; this dilatation evidently was observed in experiments by other workers [316, 17, 18], who, to all appearances, mistakenly regarded it as characteristic of cerebral edema.

Investigation of the capillary network of the cerebral cortex in rabbits after the onset of edema showed that it undergoes regular changes. The number of active capillaries (containing plasma and erythrocytes) in the cortex fell sharply; in traumatic edema their number was only one-third of the total number of capillaries in the cortex (injection of contrast material) and only just over half their number in the control experiments. Meanwhile, the lumina of the active capillaries were contracted and their diameter was actually smaller than after ligation of both carotid arteries. The changes described above in the capillary system of the brain cortex were found even in the initial stages of edema, before any marked constriction of the pial arteries had developed.

The decrease in number of active capillaries in the cerebral cortex and contraction of their lumina show that the area of their walls is reduced in edema. The extent of this decrease can be estimated from the following calculations (the figures

TABLE 1. Changes in Functional State of Parietal Cortex Capillary Network in Rabbits with Traumatic Edema. Comparison with Some Other Changes in Cerebral Circulation

Conditions of cerebral circulation	Number of active capillaries per unit volume of cerebral cortex	Diameter of capillaries (μ)
Traumatic edema	5.8 ± 0.4	5.8 ± 0.2
Ligation of both carotid arteries	8.2 ± 0.3	6.3 ± 0.14
Control	9.1 ± 0.3	6.7 ± 0.05
Injection of the cerebral vessels with contrast medium	19.1 ± 0.5	

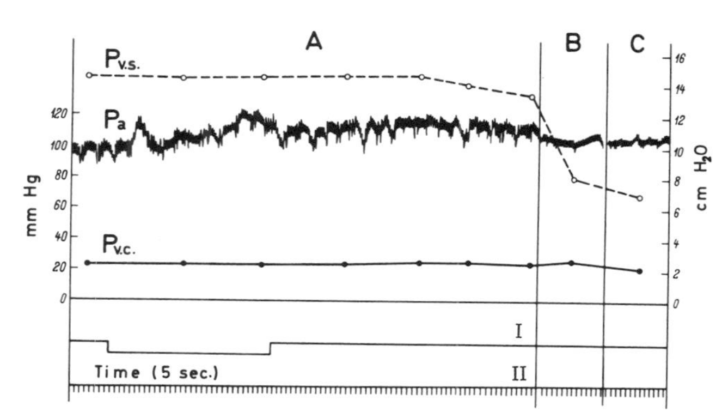

Fig. 24. Local decrease in venous pressure in sinuses of the brain during development of traumatic cerebral edema in dogs after electrical coagulation on medial surface of cerebral hemispheres [227,229]. $P_{v.s.}$, venous pressure in transverse sinus; P_a, systemic arterial pressure; $P_{v.c.}$, systemic venous pressure in the vena cava; I) marker of infliction of trauma; II) time marker (5 sec). Scale of arterial pressure on the left, scale of venous pressure on the right. A) In period of trauma; B and C) after appearance of cerebral edema (2 h 30 min and 3 h 10 min respectively after trauma).

are taken from Table 1): with a decrease in the number of active capillaries from 9.1 to 5.8 (per unit of brain volume), the area of their walls is reduced by 36%. However, the area of the walls in this 64% of the total number of active capillaries is further reduced by contraction of their lumina, from 6.7 to 5.8 μ; on account of this, the area of their walls per unit length of capillaries must be reduced by a further 13%. It thus follows that in traumatic cerebral edema the area of the capillary walls, through which transudate can be filtered from the blood into the tissues, is reduced by 44% in traumatic edema on account of a decrease in the number of active capillaries and contraction of their lumina.

Measurements of the diameter of the pial veins in dogs and rabbits have shown that these vessels were constricted in cerebral edema (the same blood vessels were measured) from 120 ± 8.1 to 93 ± 4.7 μ, i.e., on the average by 13% ($P < 0.001$). Constriction of the veins was not the result of their mechanical compression by the increased intracranial pressure, because it was observed not only when the vessels were photographed through a window (with the skull hermetically closed), but also in the region of the burr-hole when the pressure around the pial veins could not have been increased.

Measurements of the venous pressure in the brain sinuses of dogs showed that, simultaneously with the development of edema and constriction of the arterial system of the brain, this pressure fell on the average from 22 ± 2.6 to 8 ± 0.8 mm Hg, i.e., by 64% of its initial level ($P < 0.001$) (Fig. 24). This decrease in venous pressure in the brain occurred in all cases of uncomplicated edema; if, however, the cardiac activity was disturbed and the systemic venous pressure was elevated (as sometimes occurred at the end of the experiment), the blood pressure in the venous sinuses of the brain naturally showed a secondary increase.

Hence, in traumatic cerebral edema the number of active capillaries falls sharply and their lumen is contracted. There are evidently two causes of these changes. First, the decrease in intracapillary pressure taking place on account of constriction of the arterial system of the brain*; evidence of a decrease in blood pressure in the brain capillaries in edema is given by the local fall of venous pressure in the brain (which is independent of the sytemic venous pressure). Second, these changes in the capillary system in the brain in edema may also be dependent on elevation of pressure in the brain tissue resulting from swelling of glial cells and neurons surrounding the capillaries.

Consequently, the constrictor response of the internal carotid and vertebral, and also of the pial arteries, which can be regarded as characteristic of manifest edema, leads to a decrease in the blood pressure in the veins and also, evidently, in the capillaries of the brain; this, in turn, must involve a decrease in the transudation of fluid into the brain tissue, thereby limiting the development of edema. In addition, the lowering of the venous pressure must increase the reabsorption of cerebrospinal fluid and helped to lower the intracranial pressure.

*For information on the role of intracapillary pressure in the production of changes in the number of active capillaries and their lumen, see [208].

This constrictor response of the cerebral arterial system, which is seen after the development of edema, can therefore be regarded as a compensatory or protective reaction. This should not cause a significant deficiency of blood supply to the cerebral tissue, since the rate of oxygen metabolism decreases under these conditions [267].

The role of the systemic arterial pressure has been identified also during experimental traumatic cerebral edema: a sharp increase in the systemic arterial pressure led to the rapid development of edema, so that the brain after a few minutes began to protrude strongly through the burr-hole; if, however, the arterial pressure was not raised, the edema developed slowly and herniation of the brain did not reach this severity even over a period of several hours [227]. Such dependence of the magnitude of the traumatic edema on the level of the systemic arterial pressure was also observed in other studies [298]. A similar phenomenon has been observed clinically [158]; if the systemic arterial pressure rose sharply during neurosurgical operations, edema of the brain and herniation into the burr-hole developed rapidly. These results are evidently observed because the higher the intravascular pressure, the greater the degree of transudation into the brain tissue (especially under conditions of loss of autoregulation. The beneficial action of ganglion-blocking drugs on the development of edema can, perhaps, be at least partly explained by their hypotensive action: if the systemic arterial pressure is lowered to 50-60 mm Hg [62], the development of cerebral edema and swelling after neurosurgical operations on patients is less marked. The hypotensive response is evidently used by the body also under natural conditions, and it can play a protective role. For example, during the development of traumatic edema in dogs [227], a tendency was always observed for the systemic arterial pressure to fall; in cases when this pressure was not artificially stabilized, it fell at a mean rate of 19 ± 0.9 mm Hg per hour. Consequently, the systemic arterial pressure may serve as an extrinsic compensatory mechanism protecting the brain from the development of the traumatic edema.

Systemic Asphyxia

The first observations of the pial arteries in asphyxia were described in the middle of the last century by Donders [56], whose macroscopic observations showed that 10 sec after closure of the mouth and nose of a rabbit, the surface of the brain becomes red in color; in microscopic investigations Donders found that previously invisible small vessels could be seen. The volume of blood in the pial vessels again began to decrease 2 min after restoration of respiration, but it still exceeded its initial value 15 min later.

Subsequent investigations of the pial vessels in which their width was recorded by photomicrography largely confirmed the earlier observations: hitherto invisible vessels 10-20 μ in diameter appear on the brain surface; the width of these pial vessels increases considerably and this dilatation lasts 20 min after removal of the tracheal occlusion; the pial veins are constricted later than the pial arteries [148]. Dilatation of the pial arteries in rabbits was observed in asphyxia also by the present author and his co-workers [259] (Fig. 25). Although the level of the systemic arterial pressure is usually raised during asphyxia, the dilatation of the pial arteries is independent of this level, because it also takes place when the arterial pressure does not rise because of its artificial stabilization [212] (Fig. 26). This is evidence of active dilatation of the pial arteries.

The functional behavior of the major arteries of the brain during asphyxia was not studied until the end of the 1950s because their role in changes in the cerebral circulation in general had not hitherto attracted attention. It was then shown that when the trachea of a dog is occluded, the pressure in the circle of Willis falls, while the systemic arterial pressure, measured in the femoral artery, rises [407]; although these results directly indicated an increase of resistance in the major arteries of the brain, i.e., their possible constriction, no such conclusion was drawn from these observations. Simultaneous recordings of the arterial pressure in the

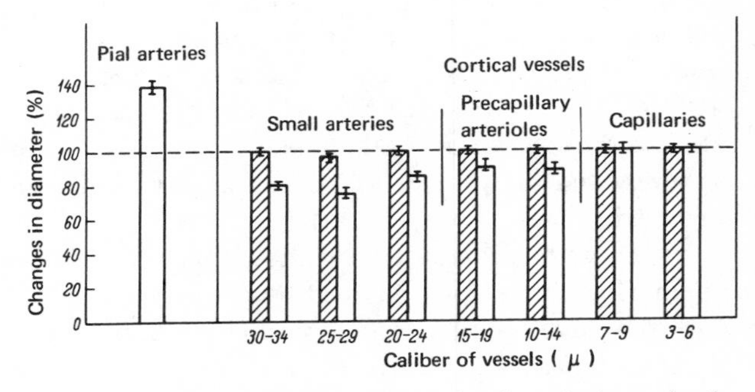

Fig. 25. Functional behavior of the pial and cortical vessels of rabbits in asphyxia. Columns denote diameter of vessels (arithmetic mean values and mean errors) in percent of initial value (pial arteries) and in percent of control values (cortical vessels). Shaded columns represent external, unshaded columns internal diameters of vessels [259].

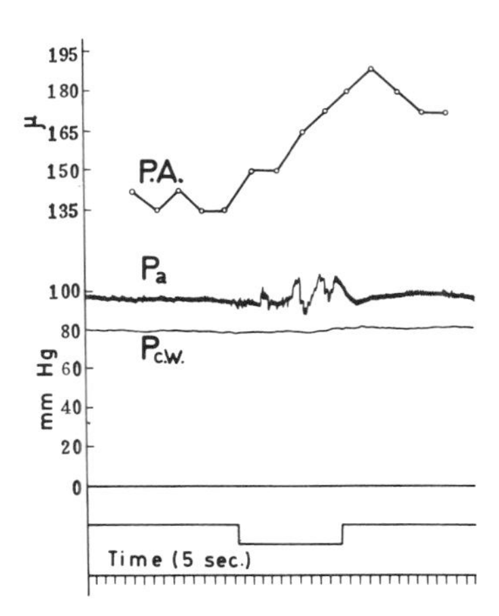

Fig. 26. Dilatation of pial arteries independently of intravascular pressure in a rabbit with asphyxia [212]. P.A., diameter of pial artery; P_a, systemic arterial pressure; $P_{C.W.}$, pressure in circle of Willis. Marker shows occlusion of trachea.

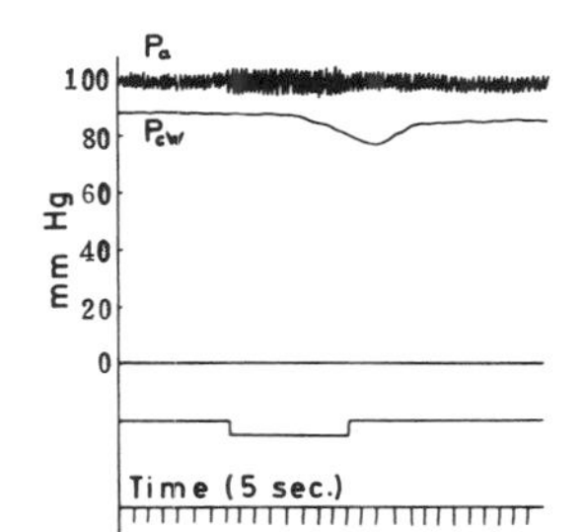

Fig. 27. Increase of resistance in major arteries of the brain during temporary tracheal occlusion. Experiment on thorax-head preparation [217]. P_a, systemic arterial pressure; $P_{C.W.}$, blood pressure in circle of Willis. Marker shows the time of tracheal occlusion.

aorta and circle of Willis made by the author [212] showed that, whereas during movement of the animal even a slight increase in systemic arterial pressure is accompanied by corresponding changes of the blood pressure in the circle of Willis, during occlusion of the trachea a much greater increase in systemic arterial pressure may sometimes be actually be accompanied by a slight decrease in the pressure in the circle of Willis, or the pressure there may rise only very slightly and after a delay. Later, to rule out the possibility of elevation of the systemic arterial pressure, similar experiments were carried out on a rabbit thorax–head preparation [217]. Under these conditions, during occlusion of the trachea, and with the pressure in the aorta unchanged, the pressure in the circle of Willis fell appreciably (Fig. 27). The difference between these pressures increased from 27 ± 4 to 33 ± 3.5 mm Hg, i.e., by 22% ($0.001 < P < 0.01$). The resistance in the major arteries of the brain was thus evidently increased, leading to a decrease of pressure in the circle of Willis. The venous pressure in the transverse sinus was nevertheless increased; this must evidently be due to a simultaneous decrease in resistance peripherally to the circle of Willis and, in particular, to dilatation of the pial arteries.

Since the pressure gradient along the major arteries of the brain does not definitely reflect their lumen during dilatation of the pial arteries, later other methods were used to assess the functional behavior of these arteries in asphyxia. For example, with the aid of a photohemotachometer, enabling quantitative measurements to be made of the volume velocity of the blood flow in large blood vessels [90], such measurements were made in the internal carotid arteries of dogs in asphyxia [241]. Assessment of the state of the internal carotid arteries on the basis of the blood flow was frequently complicated by the simultaneous elevations of the systemic arterial pressure. However, in experiments when the systemic arterial pressure remained unchanged (either naturally or because of artificial stabilization), at the beginning of asphyxia the velocity of the blood flow in the internal carotid arteries was usually increased, but later it began to flow more and more slowly, indicating constriction of these vessels, because the pial arteries located peripherally to them were widely dilated under these conditions. Constriction of both internal carotid arteries usually did not occur simultaneously. A case is illustrated in Fig. 28 in which, during occlusion of the trachea for 2 min the systemic arterial pressure did not rise; comparison of the volume velocity of the blood flow in the internal carotid artery before and after tracheal occlusion showed that it diminished from 4.5 to 0.6 ml/min, i.e., by 80%. More recently, constriction of the major arteries of the brain during asphyxia has been demonstrated on the internal carotid artery isolated *in situ*. From the time of tracheal occlusion in a dog (Fig. 29), the perfusion pressure in this artery begins to rise, and this increase continues even after the systemic arterial pressure has fallen. This increase in "tone" of the internal carotid artery during asphyxia is evidently neurogenic in its mechanism, because it was absent in experiments in which the animals were first given the sympatholytic drugs ergotamine or regitin [259].

The behavior of the cortical arteries and capillaries in asphyxia must next be discussed. Their state has been studied in rabbits in microscopic sections of the cerebral cortex fixed intravitally within 1-2 min of occlusion of the animal's trachea. Mea-

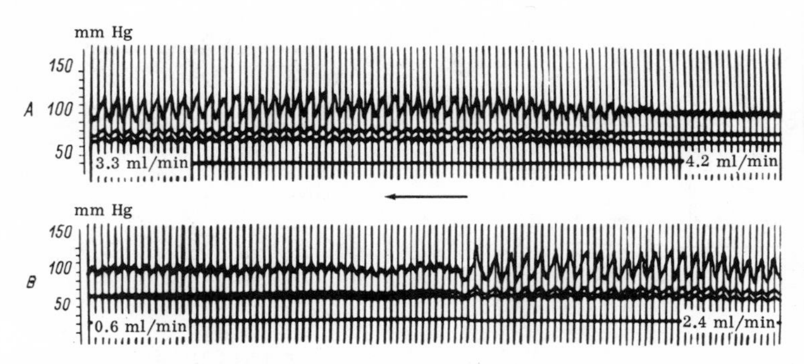

Fig. 28. Diminution of blood flow (recorded by a photohemotachometer) in internal carotid artery of a dog during temporary occlusion of the trachea (trace read from right to left) [241]. From top to bottom: systemic arterial pressure (scale on the left); two levels of pressure in differential manometer recording blood flow (absolute values of volume velocity are given below the trace); marker of tracheal occlusion. Vertical lines are time markers (1 sec). B is a direct continuation of trace A.

surement of the external and internal diameters of a large number of cortical arteries of different diameters showed that the lumen of these vessels was slightly contracted compared with the control (the differences in every case were statistcally significant), while the lumen of the capillaries remained unchanged (Fig. 25) [259]. The same results were found in animals inhaling a gas mixture containing 20% CO_2 [115].

Considering that this constriction took place in small arteries less than 40 μ in width, it could be assumed that it would not significantly increase the resistance to the blood flow because of their relatively short extent and the comparatively low velocity of the blood flow (compared with the pial arteries), and also because of the Fahraeus–Lindquist rheological phenomenon (see Chapter V). With the latest mathematical model, by means of which the vascular resistance can be determined in different parts of the arterial system of the brain from measurements of the pressures in the aorta, circle of Willis, and the venous sinuses of the brain (see Chapter I), the increase in resistance in the major arteries of the brain and in the smaller arteries located peripherally to the circle of Willis has been calculated in dogs with asphyxia (Fig. 30). These

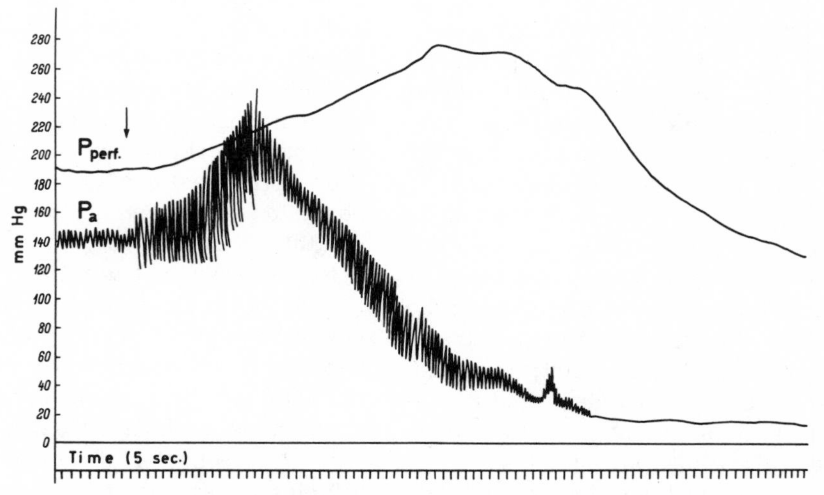

Fig. 29. Increase of resistance in internal carotid artery of a dog, isolated in situ during asphyxia [259]. $P_{perf.}$, perfusion pressure in internal carotid artery; P_a, systemic arterial pressure. Arrow indicates time of occlusion of trachea, after which perfusion pressure began to rise, indicating a constriction of this artery.

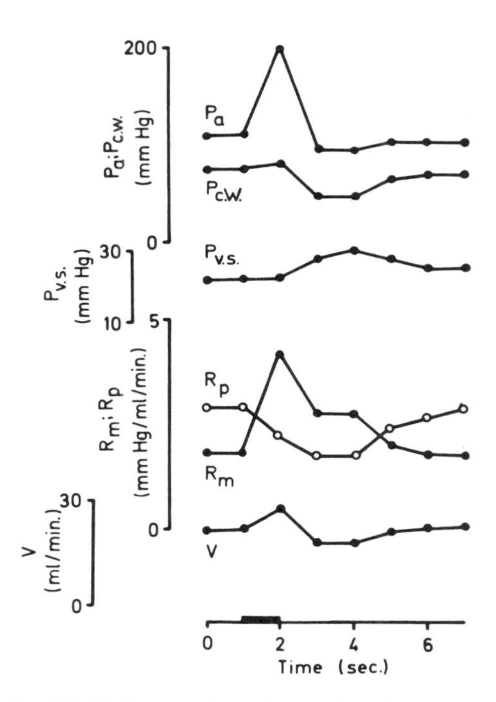

Fig. 30. Resistances in major arteries of the brain (R_m) and in small arteries peripheral to the circle of Willis (R_p) calculated by means of a mathematical model from pressures recorded in physiological experiments on dogs in the aorta (P_a), circle of Willis (P_{cW}), and venous sinuses of the brain in asphyxia due to mechanical occlusion of the tracheotomy tube. Volume velocity of blood flow calculated from data thus obtained [248].

results are in full agreement with those of previously cited investigations of all these vessels using other methods.

Despite the constriction of the major arteries of the brain and the slight constriction of the cortical arteries taking place during asphyxia, the dilatation of the pial arteries produces a decrease in the cerebrovascular resistance (in about 50% of all experiments by the present author) that the blood flow into the brain is increased in asphyxia even before the systemic arterial pressure has begun to rise. This earlier increase in the cerebral blood flow occurred in dogs on the average 35 ± 5.3 sec before the beginning of elevation of the systemic arterial pressure, and an increase in the blood volume in the brain has also been observed without any increase in the systemic arterial pressure in asphyxia [285].

Postischemic States

Postischemic states of the brain regularly develop when the cerebral circulation is interrupted or significantly decreased for a short time and then restored. Some authors assume that cerebral edema usually develops in postischemic states of the brain, since histological investigations of the brain of dogs surviving after clinical death usually revealed all the evidence of cerebral edema and swelling: dilatation of the cerebral ventricles, perivascular zones of translucency, swelling of nerve cells, vacuolation of their cytoplasm, and so on [2, 329, 386] However, it was then found that the content of water in the brain tissue was not increased in the majority of experimental animals surviving after clinical death caused by mechanical asphyxia (occlusion of the trachea); it is therefore open to question whether cerebral edema really is a regular sequel to any postischemic state of the brain [99, 293].

The functional behavior of different brain vessels during the postischemic state has been studied in rabbits [214]. Bleeding from the abdominal aorta resulted in a drop of the systemic arterial pressure and stoppage of the cerebral circulation, and some 1-2 min later blood was injected back into the artery toward the heart. The systemic arterial pressure was thus restored to its original level. The pressure recorded simultaneously in the circle of Willis also began to rise, but as is shown in Fig. 31, when the original pressure in the aorta was fully restored, the pressure in the circle of Willis was still far below its original level. The difference between the pressures in the aorta and circle of Willis, which may reflect the resistance in the major arteries of the brain, was increased on the average from 13 ± 2 to 36 ± 3.6 mm Hg, i.e., by 177% ($P < 0.001$). This could indicate marked constriction of the internal carotid and vertebral arteries. Restoration of the initial difference between these pressures took place gradually, on the average 20-30 min after the beginning of intra-arterial injection of blood.

After temporary interruption of the circulation in the brain a similar phenomenon was observed in dogs. For instance, after removal of temporary occlusion of the aorta [231], the pressure difference in the aorta and circle of Willis (the systemic arterial pressure remaining almost the same) rose from 25 ± 2 to 40 ± 2.5 mm Hg, i.e., by 60% ($P < 0.001$). Consequently, the postischemic state of the dog's brain seems also to be accompanied by a marked increase of resistance in the major arteries of the brain. The same result was observed when the circulation in the dog's brain was interrupted by a temporary increase of intracranial pressure up to the level of the blood pressure in the circle of Willis [230]. Evidence of a sharp decrease in, or the total cessation of, the circulation

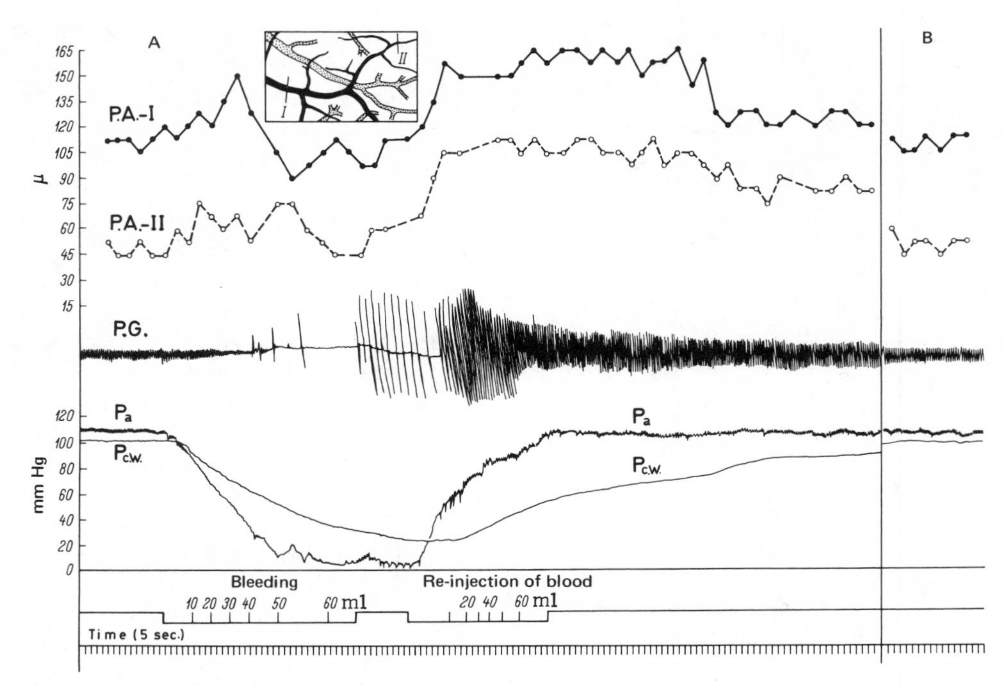

Fig. 31. Dilatation of pial arteries and pressure gradient increase in major arteries of the brain after temporary cerebral ischemia produced by bleeding from the abdominal aorta [214]. P.A.(I), large and P.A.(II), small pial arteries (these vessels are shown diagrammatically above); P.G., pneumogram; P_a, systemic arterial pressure; $P_{c.w.}$, pressure in circle of Willis. The marker shows time of bleeding and re-injection of blood; B, 20 min after A.

of blood in the brain under these conditions was given by the sharp decrease in amplitude of spontaneous cortical electrical activity (Fig. 32). When the circulation in the brain was restored and the systemic arterial pressure maintained at its original level (it usually had to be stabilized artificially), the difference between the pressures in the aorta and circle of Willis was increased on the average from 33 ± 2 to 54 ± 2 mm Hg, i.e., by 64% ($P < 0.001$).

Consequently, an increase of the pressure gradient in the major arteries of the brain after cerebral ischemia is regularly observed under a variety of experimental conditions. However, an increase of resistance alone in this case would be insufficient evidence of active constriction of these arteries, for the pial arteries located at the periphery were dilated under these same conditions (see below), and consequently, the resistance in them was evidently reduced. The results of experiments using different methods of investigation are therefore important evidence of active constriction of the system of major arteries of the brain under these conditions. Recent experiments using resistography of the internal carotid arteries, isolated *in situ*, have yielded direct evidence of the constriction and increase in resistance of these vessels during the development of postischemic cerebral edema (Fig. 33). Since an increase in the resistance of the major arteries of the brain could result in a decrease in the intracapillary pressure within the brain, the vasoconstriction of these arteries might be a protective mechanism preventing the development of cerebral edema [214, 332, 181].

The functional behavior of the pial arteries in postischemic states of the brain was investigated by serial photomicrography. When the circulation in the brain was restored (after interruption for 1 or 2 min) the pial arteries of the rabbit dilated considerably, and the magnitude of the dilator response was particularly great in the case of the small arteries (Fig. 31). Arteries whose initial diameter was smaller than 75 mm were dilated on the average by 69 ± 10%, and wider arteries by 29 ± 2.2% (Fig. 34). This was undoubtedly an active response of the pial arteries, because the level of the systemic arterial pressure remained the same under these circumstances as before bleeding, while the major arteries of the brain, as shown above, actually became constricted during this period [214]. Later the pial arteries began to constrict gradu-

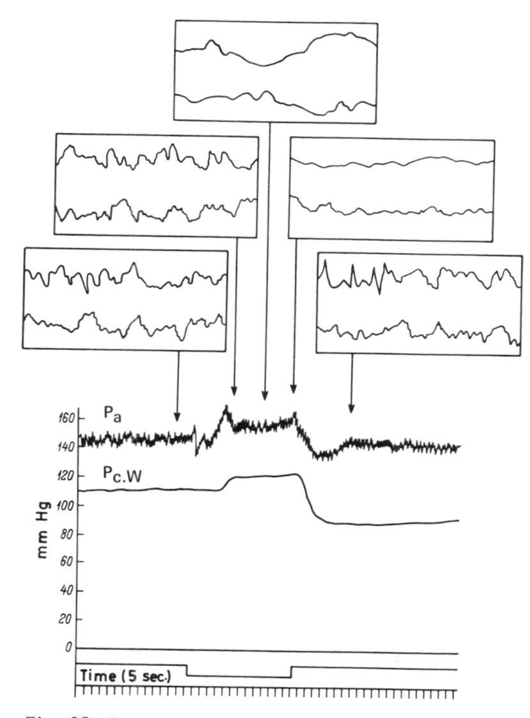

Fig. 32. Increase in pressure gradient in major arteries of the dog's brain after a temporary increase of intracranial pressure to 125 mm Hg [230]. EEG patterns at various times of the experiment shown within rectangles. P_a, systemic arterial pressure; $P_{c.W.}$, pressure in circle of Willis. Marker shows time of elevation of intracranial pressure.

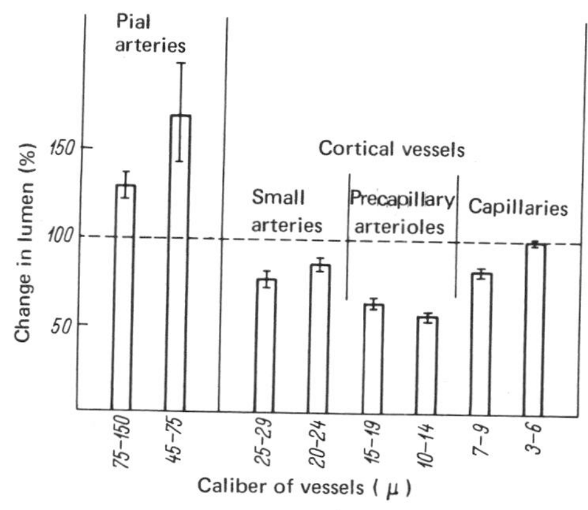

Fig. 34. Functional behavior of the pial and cortical vessels of different caliber in postischemic states of the brain (in rabbits). Columns denote diameter of vascular lumen (arithmetic means and standard deviations) in percent of initial value (pial arteries), and in percent of control values (cortical arteries) [237].

ally, but as a rule this process did not take place parallel with restoration of the original pressure in the circle of Willis. This was further evidence that dilatation of the pial arteries and the increase of resistance in the major arteries of the brain were not interconnected as cause and effect.

Basically similar results were obtained in experiments by other researchers [379] on monkeys; after temporary occlusion of both internal carotid arteries, the systemic arterial pressure rose while the pressure in the large branches of

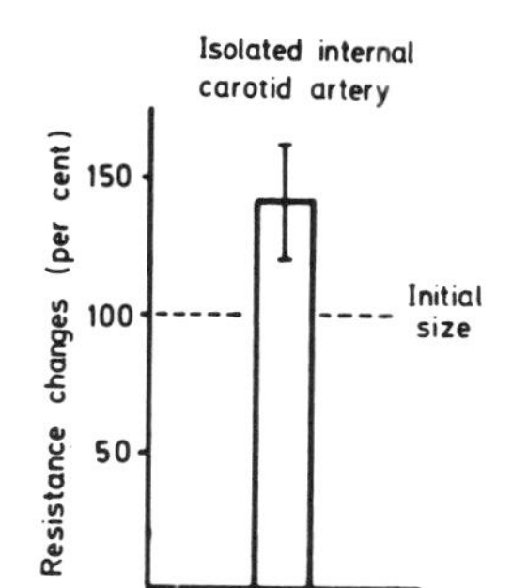

Fig. 33. Significant increase in resistance of internal carotid artery of a dog, isolated in situ, after development of postischemic cerebral edema.

the pial arteries remained unchanged; this indicated an increase of resistance along the course of the major arterial trunks and other large arteries of the brain. Meanwhile the blood flow in the cerebral cortex (recorded by means of thermistors) was increased, possibly because of a decrease in resistance in the small pial arteries (which must have been dilated under these conditions) and, possibly, in the intracerebral vessels (for details of the state of these vessels under these circumstances, see below).

Even a transient (lasting a few minutes) interruption of the circulation to the brain gives rise to prolonged metabolic changes characteristic of a deficient blood supply in it. These changes may persist even after restoration of the circulation [287, 86, 233]. The dilatation of the pial arteries described above is evidently a manifestation of postischemic (reactive) hyperemia, i.e., a compensatory reaction aimed at eliminating the consequences of the deficient blood supply to the brain.

The functional behavior of small arteries and arterioles in the depth of the cerebral cortex during the development of postischemic states of the brain has also been studied [234, 246, 237]. The principle of the method used was as follows: during ischemia lasting 1 or 2 min, and at various times after restoration of the circulation in the brain, the walls of blood vessels were fixed intravitally, and their state was then studied in brain sections (details of the method are given in Chapter II). In this way the dy-

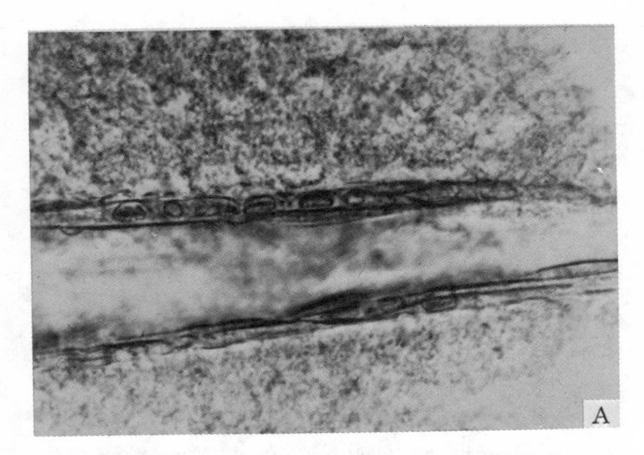

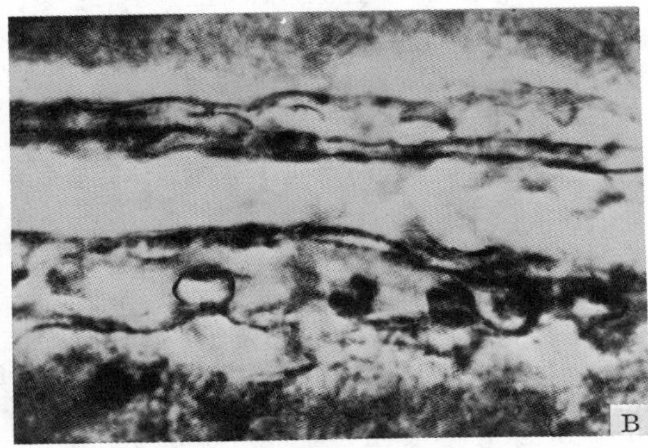

Fig. 35. Changes in walls of a cortical artery in ischemia: separation of vessel wall into layers, with erythrocytes escaping by diapedesis into the intramural space. Photomicrographs, unretouched, 400X. A) control; B) ischemia.

namics of changes in diameter and structure of the walls of the cerebral vessels and surrounding tissue could be studied during the development of postischemic states of the brain. The investigations showed that the principal characteristic morphological changes developing actually in the period of ischemia are swelling of the structural elements of the walls of the intracerebral arteries and separation into layers of the connective-tissue structures of the vessel walls (Fig. 35), as a result of which they become thickened. The external diameter was not appreciably changed along the course of the cortical vessels, but the internal diameter was regularly reduced, especially in the precapillary arterioles. Differences from the control were in all cases statistically significant (Fig. 34). It is difficult as yet to be specific regarding the character of the effect of this narrowing of the lumen of the cortical arteries on the vascular resistance. The possibility is not ruled out that a very slight constriction of such small cortical arteries (40 μ and less) does not appreciably increase the resistance to the blood flow and does not prevent an increase in blood supply to the cerebral cortex when this is deficient (see Chapter V). However, in the presence of marked constriction of the small vessels in the brain substance, the cerebrovascular resistance in the corresponding regions could increase very considerably and the circulation in them is not restored in the postischemic state [4, 42, 163]. An increase in the relative viscosity of the blood evidently also plays an important role in increasing the cerebrovascular resistance under these conditions. It has been shown, for example, that under conditions of this type aggregation of the blood platelets begins to take place, hindering its flow along the small vessels [246].

The increase in resistance developing in the major arteries of the brain in postischemic states, together with marked constriction of the intracerebral arteries and arterioles, and also with an increase in the relative viscosity of the blood, may increase the total cerebrovascular resistance to such an extent that the blood flow in the brain is severely reduced. Recordings of the blood flow in the internal carotid artery in monkeys showed that during spontaneous restoration of the systemic arterial pressure after severe hemorrhage, the blood flow in this artery was diminished, and in the opinion of the workers concerned, this indicated constriction of these vessels [332]. Measurements of the blood flow in the internal carotid artery of dogs showed that after clinical death it returns to normal only 5-6 min or longer after recovery of the systemic arterial pressure [181]. So far as the volume velocity of the blood flow in the cerebral cortex, recorded by Gibbs' needles in cats under the same experimental conditions (bleeding and subsequent intra-arterial injection of blood), is concerned, this remained below its original level for 10-20 min [181, 182]. Similar results were found when the oxygen tension in the cortex was measured polarographically: recovery of the initial oxygen tension frequently occurred much later than in other organs, for example, the liver [182, 259]. All these experimental data, obtained in recent years, indicate that in the postischemic state the blood supply to the brain may be reduced despite restoration of the normal level of the systemic arterial pressure and dilatation of the pial arteries lying peripherally to the circle of Willis.

Hence, during the development of the postischemic state of the brain, different parts of its arterial system behave differently: a) the major arteries of the brain (internal carotid and vetebral arteries) are constricted, presumably to compensate for the development of edema or other disorders in the brain, b) the pial arteries (especially the small arteries) are dilated, in all probability to compensate for the deficiency of blood supply to the brain tissue, and c) the lumen of the intracerebral arteries is constricted. In this way the different manifestations of functional behavior of these three divisions of the cerebral arterial system are brought about.

Because the above changes in the lumen of different parts of the arterial system of the brain take place in different directions, the intensity of the circulation in it may vary unequally: it may be reduced (evidently when constriction of the major arteries of the brain or of the intracerebral arteries and arterioles is predominant), it may be increased (when a decrease in resistance in the pial arteries is predominant) and, finally, it may remain unchanged (because the changes in resistance in the different parts of the cerebral arterial system cancel each other out).

Increased Activity of the Cerebral Cortex

The activity of the nervous structures of the brain is closely linked with changes in metabolism, and an adequate blood supply is therefore necessary [365]. It has been shown that under ordinary conditions the blood supply to the brain is about twice that required to satisfy the metabolic needs of its tissue elements [343], but in the presence of a marked increase in activity of the brain tissues the circulation of blood in the brain is also increased. This view was originally put forward as long ago as at the end of the last century, and it was confirmed, beginning in the 1930s, by many workers using different methods of increasing brain activity and different methods of recording the circulation in it. In response to adequate stimulation of the receptors of the eye, an increased circulation in the optic tract, in the intermediate nuclei, and in the cortical receptor areas was demonstrated by several methods: by recording the temperature of the brain tissue with thermocouples [92, 349] and thermistors [45] or thermoelectric detectors [187], by electroplethysmography [5, 16], and also by the accumulation of an inert radioactive gas in the brain tissue [366]. Increased cortical activity, in the form of "desynchronization" of the electrocorticogram, developing in response to stimulation of the mesencephalic reticular formation, is accompanied by an increase in the cortical circulation; this was shown originally by direct observations on the pial vessels under the microscope [120], and later by recording the outflow of blood from the sagittal venous sinus draining blood from the corresponding area of the cortex [121, 127]. Further, the same effect was demonstrated by recording the cerebral blood flow by a thermoelectric technique [166], as well as recording the blood outflow through the internal jugular vein with an electromagnetic flowmeter [268]. A similar increase of the circulation in the cortex was observed also in waking cats, when, besides changes in cortical electrical activity, the important role of the animals' behavior (movements, orienting reaction) was observed [136]. The same result was observed in the spinal cord of rabbits during stimulation of peripheral nerves [70]. The increase in blood supply to the corresponding cortical areas described in response to an increase in their functional activity is of great importance for the maintenance of normal metabolism. Polarographic investigations have shown that at the beginning of a period of increased cortical activity (during adequate stimulation of receptors or electrical stimulation of the mesencephalon and diencephalon), the oxygen tension in the brain falls, but very soon, because of the increased circulation, it not only recovers but actually exceeds its original level [263, 124]. An increase of oxygen consumption in the cerebral cortex with augmented activity has also been demonstrated in recent studies [268].

The fact that the circulation is increased in an area of cortex whose activity is considerably intensified has thus been demonstrated by many investigations. However, none of these investigations published before 1960 considered the problem of which of the brain vessels are responsible for these changes in the circulation of the blood. Therefore the physiological mechanism of this vasodilatation could not be adequately studied either. All that has been proved so far is that any increase in circulation in the brain which depends on the degree of its activity is due to dilatation of vessels of the brain itself, and can take place even if the level of the systemic arterial pressure is stabilized and does not itself increase.

Correlation between the functional behavior of different vascular mechanisms and activity of the brain has been studied by the writer and his coworkers over the last decade in experiments on rabbits, either unanesthetized or lightly anesthetized with urethane. An increase in activity in the parietal cortex was evoked by local application of 0.5-

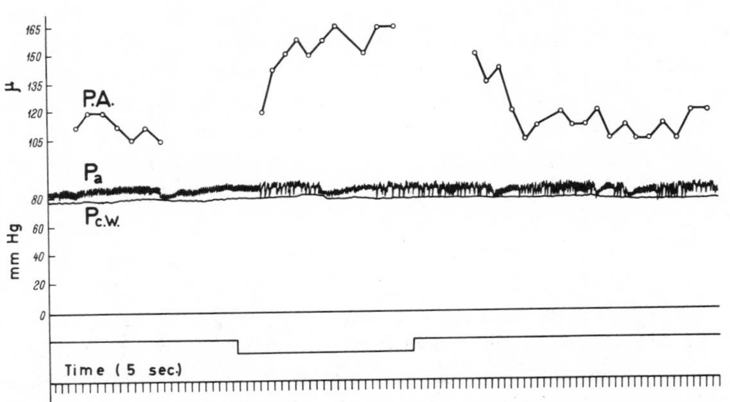

Fig. 36. Dilatation of pial arteries independent of systemic arterial pressure and of state of the major arteries of the brain, during application of strychnine to the brain surface [212]. P.A., diameter of pial arteries, P_a, arterial pressure in aorta, $P_{c.W.}$, pressure in circle of Willis. The marker shows the time of application of strychnine.

1.0% strychnine solution in isotonic saline to the brain surface. Even in unanesthetized animals the systemic arterial pressure remained unchanged, so that it was unnecessary to use artificial stabilization. After application of strychnine to the parietal cortex (Fig. 36), the pial arteries became sharply dilated, but the blood pressure in the aorta and in the circle of Willis remained unchanged; this indicates that the resistance in the major arteries of the brain, and consequently their lumen, were unchanged [212]. A local increase in the circulation in the brain associated with increased activity of its neurons can therefore take place without any appreciable changes in the lumen of the internal carotid and vertebral arteries. At the same time, the pial arteries in the region of local application of strychnine were dilated, and by serial photomicrography it was possible to examine the whole course of changes in the width of these vessels. The smaller the caliber of the pial arteries, the greater was the degree of their dilatation; arteries with an initial diameter smaller than 75 μ, for instance, dilated twice as much as wider vessels (Fig. 37). The areas of action of strychnine, of changes in electrical activity, and of dilatation of the pial arteries approximately coincided.

The next problem to consider is whether in these experiments the increased blood supply is in fact dependent on the functional activity of the cortex, or whether dilatation of the pial arteries is due to direct action of strychnine on them. This last possibility was ruled out experimentally. First, vasodilatation occurred only in those experiments in which corresponding changes were found in the electrocorticogram. After the direct application of 10% tetraethylammonium bromide (which blocks nicotine-like cholinergic receptors in the cortex itself but does not affect muscarine-like cholinergic receptors in the vessel walls [13]) to the brain surface, both the changes in the electrocorticograms evoked by strychnine and the dilatation of the pial arteries were diminished (Table 2). Second, during the direct action of strychnine on the pial arteries, not only were they not dilated, but sometimes they actually were constricted (like those in other organs). In some experiments, for instance, these arteries were seen to be slightly constricted during the period of strychnine application and dilated im-

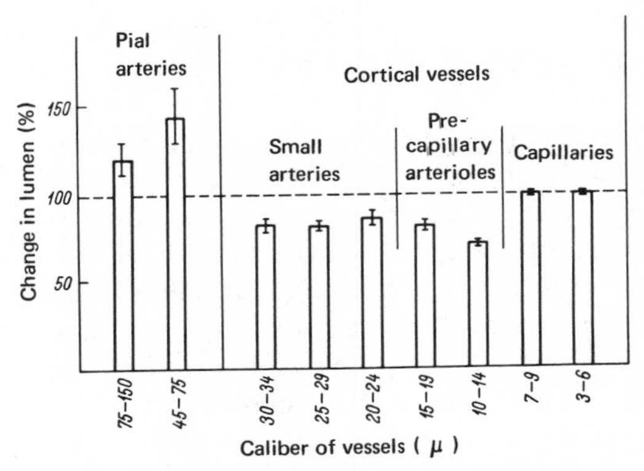

Fig. 37. Functional behavior of the pial and cortical vessels of different caliber during stimulation of cortical activity after local application of 0.5% strychnine (rabbits). Columns denote diameter of vascular lumen (arithmetic means and standard deviation) in % of initial value (pial arteries) and in % of control values (cortical vessels) [237].

TABLE 2. Changes in Electrocorticogram and Reaction of Pial Arteries during Local Application of Strychnine before and after Blocking of Nicotine-like Cholinergic Receptors in the Cerebral Cortex with 10% Tetraethylammonium Bromide (TEA)

Indices studied	Control ($M \pm \sigma$)	Against background of action of TEA bromide ($M \pm \sigma$)	Index of significance of difference (P)
Increase in amplitude of electrocorticogram (in % of initial)	146 ± 43.8	106 ± 3	< 0.001
Dilatation of pial arteries (in % of initial diameter)	139 ± 11.6	120 ± 10.6	< 0.01 and > 0.001

mediately after its removal (while the electrocorticogram continued to be changed); on the other hand, after microsurgical separation of the vessel from the pia mater over a distance of a few millimeters and introduction of a thin glass disc beneath it, the artery did not react or even constricted in response to the application of strychnine to it [218]. Consequently, dilatation of the pial arteries is not dependent on the direct action of strychnine on them, but on the primary intensification of cortical activity and subsequent influences from the cortex on the walls of these vessels.

The temporal correlations between the development of changes in the electrocorticogram and dilatation of the pial arteries also were studied [250]. After application of strychnine to the cortex (Fig. 37), the pial arteries dilate until distinct changes appeared in the spontaneous electrical activity, and they started to contract when the amplitude of the electrocorticogram was still increasing and was showing signs of paroxysmal discharges. The results of statistical analysis of the results of all (64) experiments were as follows: dilatation of the pial arteries reached a maximum after 60 ± 6.7 sec; at this time the amplitude of the electrocorticogram was only 80 ± 4% of its maximum (the time of appearance of paroxysmal discharges is less constant in rabbits than, for example, in cats). The maximum of vasodilatation occurred 44 ± 9.8 sec before the maximum of amplitude of the electrocorticogram, and by the time that the electrocorticogram reached its maximum, the pial arteries had already begun to constrict; their diameter then was 83 ± 1.6% of its previous maximum.

Investigation of the capillary networks (see Chapter I) in the rabbit cerebral cortex after intravital fixation by application of 20% formalin solution in 96% alcohol to the brain surface [206] showed that, simultaneously with dilatation of the pial arteries, after application of strychnine the capillary circulation increases in the corresponding cortical areas. The number of active capillaries in the cortex was about 50% greater than in the contralateral (control) hemisphere (Table 3). The increase in number of active capillaries (in this case, evidently, conversion of plasma-filled capillaries into active [208]) was partly due to an increase in the number of erythrocytes in the blood entering the corresponding capillary network from the dilated pial arteries. This increase was discovered by intravital fixation of the pia mater following the application of strychnine to the corresponding part of the brain surface [216]. In more recent investigations, in which the vessel walls were fixed intravitally by perfusing the vascular system at different times after local application of 0.5-1% strychnine solution to the cortical surface of unanesthetized rabbits, and the cortical vessels were then examined in histological sections, the state of vascular behavior could be studied under those conditions [235, 244]. These experiments showed that, soon after application of strychnine (before the corresponding changes appeared in the electrocorticogram), characteristic and gradually increasing changes took place in these vessels. The external diameter of the cortical arteries was not increased but, on the contrary, it showed a tendency to decrease. At the same time the internal diameter and, consequently, the lumen of the small cortical arteries and, in particular, the

TABLE 3. Number of Active Capillaries (Open and Filled with Erythrocytes and Blood Plasma) per Unit Volume of Parietal Cortex of Rabbits 5 min after Application of 1% Strychnine

Cortical area studied	Number of fields of vision of microscope examined	Number of active capillaries	Index of significance of difference (P)
Region of application of strychnine	40	13.3 ± 0.5	
Control: symmetrically opposite area of cortex	50	9.1 ± 0.35	< 0.001

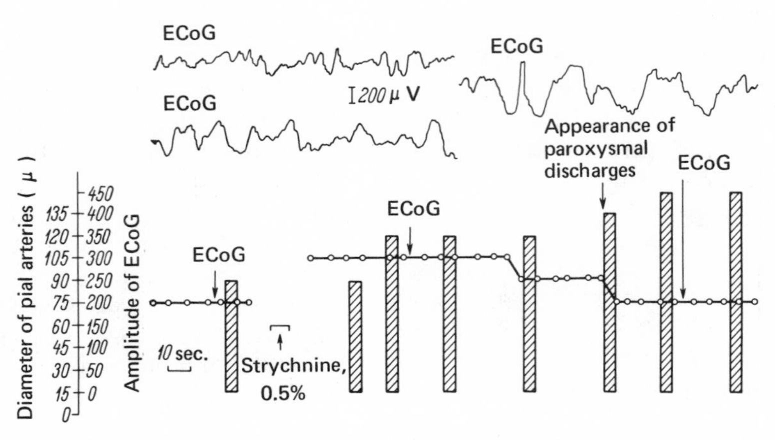

Fig. 38. Relationship between diameter of pial arteries (horizontal line) and changes in amplitude of electrocortigogram after application of 0.5% strychnine to the rabbit cerebral cortex. Specimens of the electrocorticogram are given above [250]. Explanation in text.

arterioles was regularly diminished (Fig. 38). If the pial arteries are dilated, a very slight constriction of the lumen of the small cortical arteries 10-40 μ in diameter evidently does not reduce the intensity of the capillary circulation in the corresponding cortical area (because of their shorter length and the slower blood flow in them, and also because of the increased fluidity of the blood in these vessels resulting from the Fahraeus–Lindqvist effect (for details see Chapter V). The intensity of the circulation in the cerebral cortex of cats was investigated by the krypton clearance technique [123]. These experiments showed [125, 244] that in the region of application of strychnine the maximal increase in blood flow averaged 45% of the initial value (from 1.2 to 1.76 ml/g tissue/min on the average). This maxi-

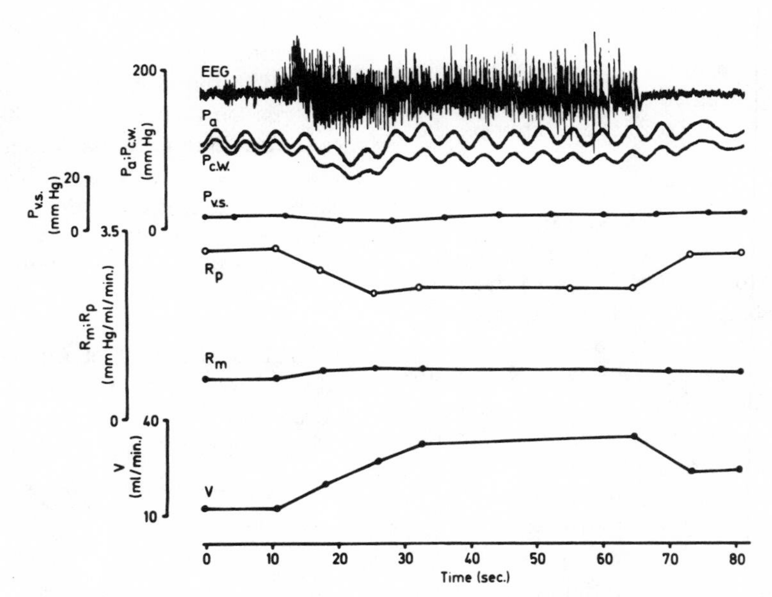

Fig. 39. Resistances in major arteries of brain (R_m) and in small arteries peripherally to circle of Willis (R_p) calculated by means of the mathematical model from pressures recorded in physiological experiments on dogs in aorta (P_a), circle of Willis (P_{cW}) and venous sinuses of the brain (P_{vs}) on the appearance of paroxysmal electrical activity (EEG) induced by intra-arterial injection of ten mg strychnine. Volume velocity of blood flow calculated from results thus obtained (experiments by Mchedlishvili, Mitagvariya, and Ormotsadze).

mal increase of the cortical circulation usually occurred 6-10 min after the application of strychnine, and thereafter the intensity began to decrease.

Recent determinations of the resistance in the major arteries of the brain and in vessels located peripherally to the circle of Willis by the use of the mathematical model (see Chapter I) have shown (Fig. 39) that in dogs the resistance in the pial and cortical arteries is substantially reduced after intra-arterial injection of strychnine, while in the major arteries it is slightly increased, perhaps either through the direct action of strychnine on these vessels or as a result of reflex overfilling of the cerebral vessels with blood.

It can be concluded from all these observations that when activity of the cerebral cortex is stimulated, its blood supply is increased mainly through dilatation of the pial arteries, and that neither the internal carotid nor the vertebral arteries react. This is further evidence that in the vascular system of the brain, it is the pial arteries which are responsible for changes in the cerebral circulation associated with increased activity of the brain tissue. The slight contraction of the lumen of the cortical arteries occurring at the same time may actually not prevent the increased blood flow in the corresponding area of cortex.

Ischemia of the Cerebral Cortex Resulting from Occlusion of the Pial Arteries

When from 3 to 6 main trunks of the pial arteries carrying blood into the parietal cortex were occluded by diathermy coagulation, the inflow of blood along other arteries located in the neighborhood quickly increased [255]. In the experiment whose results are given in Table 4, for instance, the velocity of inflow of blood was almost trebled. Since the blood pressure in the aorta and in the circle of Willis remained unchanged under these circumstances (Fig. 40B), this effect could only be due to dilatation of arteries located peripherally to the circle of Willis. This compensatory reaction of the pial arteries facilitated a collateral blood supply and was able to prevent the development of cortical ischemia, as shown by the absence of hypoxic changes in the electrocortigram (Fig. 40B).

After occlusion of all branches along which blood could reach the parietal region over the brain surface, ischemia developed in the cortex. The velocity of the inflow of blood from the circle of Willis into the pial arteries in the parietal region fell sharply. For instance, in the experiment whose results are given in Table 4, it was reduced by more than four-fifths compared with those obtained initially. At the same time, a retrograde blood flow appeared in the veins on the brain surface, and the blood in them became arterial in color. (This phenomenon is evidently compensatory, but its hemodynamic mechanism is not yeat clear.) The presence of ischemia in the parietal cortex was indicated by the following observations. First, *in vivo* microscopic investigations revealed marked slowing, or actually complete arrest, of the blood flow in the pial arteries, which became cyanotic in color as if the vessels contained venous blood. Second, when trypan blue (1%, 1 ml/kg body weight) was injected into the blood stream, it penetrated into the vessels of the whole brain except the parietal cortex, where the pial arteries had previously been occluded. Third, evidence of a considerable deficiency of blood supply was given by characteristic changes in the electrocorticogram: to begin with slow waves appeared while fast waves were weakened, but in cases of more marked ischemia, spontaneous electrical activity was sharply reduced or disappeared completely; in the contralateral hemisphere no significant changes were observed in the electrocorticogram (Fig. 40). Similar changes in the microcirculation – in particular a decrease in the velocity of blood flow, aggregation of erythro-

TABLE 4. Changes in Velocity of Inflow of Blood from the Circle of Willis into the Parietal Cortex of a Rabbit after Occlusion of the Pial Arteries at the Edges of the Burr-Hole ($P < 0.001$)

	Initial state	Immediately after occlusion of four main branches	Immediately after occlusion of all arteries	17 min later
Mean time of inflow of blood from circle of Willis into pial artery (in sec)	1.7 ± 0.04	0.6 ± 0.06	8.8 ± 0.2	5.6 ± 0.17
Mean velocity of inflow of blood from circle of Willis into pial artery (mm/sec)	13	36.6	2.5	3.9

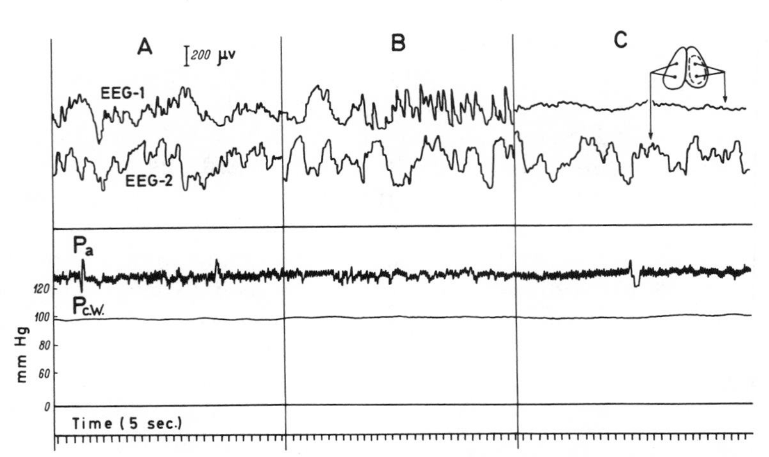

Fig. 40. Cortical electrical activity, systemic arterial pressure, and pressure gradient in major arteries of the brain during development of a focus of ischemia in the parietal cortex on the right side [255]. EEG-1 and EEG-2, patterns of electrocorticograms (location of electrodes indicated on diagram in top right corner; P_a, systemic arterial pressure; $P_{c.W.}$, blood pressure in circle of Willis. A) before, B) after occlusion of some pial arteries; C) after occlusion of all pial arteries and onset of ischemia.

cytes, etc. – on the brain surface have recently been observed also by other researchers [401] after occlusion of the middle cerebral artery in monkeys and cats.

When such a focus of ischemia appeared in the parietal cortex of rabbits, no changes were found in the systemic arterial pressure; the blood pressure in the circle of Willis also remained unchanged (Fig. 39). It may therefore be assumed that the resistance in the major arteries of the brain remained unchanged. Since the experiments were carried out on unanesthetized animals, the possibility of suppression of reflex or humoral influences on these blood vessels was ruled out. Again, it follows that during local ischemia of the cortex neither the systemic arterial pressure nor the major arteries of the brain participate in the mechanism of regulation of the cerebral circulation, which maintains an adequate blood supply to the cerebral cortex in accordance with its metabolic demands. The foregoing remarks show that this kind of regulation of the inflow of blood into the cerebral tissue is mainly effected by changes in the diameter of the pial arteries.

The view was held, from the 19th century until the last decade, that when the blood supply to the brain becomes insufficient, this is always accompanied by elevation of the systemic arterial pressure. Since the time of Magendie [195] it has been known that compression of the carotid arteries increases the heart rate and elevates the arterial pressure; these results were considered to be due to influences from brain centers experiencing an insufficient blood supply. However, it was later discovered that such hypertensive effects are due to a reflex in response to a drop in pressure in the area of the carotid baroreceptors [6, 109, 110, 153]. The pressor response is similar if the intracranial pressure rises sharply, and in this case also it was thought to be a result of deficiency of the blood supply to the brain tissue [48, 404, 144]. Later work showed, however, that the pressor response is also reflex in origin, arising to stimulation of the baroreceptors inside the skull [327, 328]. Evidence against the conclusion that elevation of the systemic arterial pressure under the conditions described is the result of an insufficient blood supply to the brain is also provided by experiments in which the deficiency of blood supply to the brain tissue was brought about by ligation of the middle cerebral artery [159, 401] and by occlusion of the cranial vena cava [232]. Only when complete ischemia was produced in that part of the medulla where the vasomotor center is located (by careful occlusion of the corresponding arteries) was a small increase (14 mm Hg) of the systemic arterial pressure observed [148]. This was later confirmed by a different method: in cases of embolism of blood vessels of the forebrain and hemisphere, severe ischemia, manifested by typical changes in the electroencephalogram developed, yet the systemic arterial pressure was not elevated; it was raised only in cases when arteries of the medulla were blocked by emboli [385].

Consequently, all the available experimental data show that insufficiency of the blood supply to various parts of the brain (except the medulla) does not cause elevation of the systemic arterial pressure. The opposite conclusions, which were drawn initially from experiments in which the common carotid arteries were compressed and the intracranial pressure was raised, subsequently proved groundless, because the arterial pressure was raised in such cases as a result of reflexes from the carotid sinus or intracranial baroreceptors. Moreover, if such a mechanism of regulation of the cerebral circulation really existed, the level of the systemic arterial pressure would rise every time the blood supply to any part of the brain became insufficient. Without mentioning the pointlessness of such a method of control (simultaneous changes in the blood supply of other organs), its existence, as was mentioned above, has not been proved experimentally.

Collateral Blood Supply

Compensation of a deficiency of blood supply to the cerebral hemispheres following occlusion of one of the internal carotid arteries can take place through the collateral inflow of blood in the region of the circle of Willis from other major arteries of the brain. In mammals, the brain, unlike all other organs of the body is supplied with blood by four major arteries connected in parallel: the paired internal carotid and vertebral arteries. If the system of major arteries to the brain is examined at the various levels of phylogenetic development, it becomes clear that these unique structural features have arisen in vertebrates in the course of evolution [93, 132]. For example, in fishes, amphibians, reptiles, and birds the brain is supplied principally by the two carotid arteries, and the circle of Willis, as such, is absent. In certain mammals (in particular, cats) the internal carotid arteries are obliterated and their functions taken over by anastomoses between branches of the external carotid artery and the circle of Willis; in dogs an extensive arterial anastomosis is present between the internal carotid and external ophthalmic arteries. The reason for the appearance of these special types of blood supply to the brain, which have disappeared in the subsequent stages of evolution (in monkeys and in man), is not yet clear.

Although, near the base of the brain, its major arteries are joined to form the circle of Willis, under ordinary conditions the blood in it is not mixed; from each major trunk the blood enters only the corresponding cerebral vessels of the ipsilateral side: the internal carotid arteries supply the cerebral hemispheres, and the vertebral arteries supply mainly the cerebellum and medulla. This has been demonstrated by injecting radio-opaque or radioactive substances and dyes into the major arteries to the brain [341, 115, 112]. The absence of mixing of the blood in the region of the circle of Willis is explained by the fact that under normal conditions the pressure in the end of all major arteries to the brain is about equal, so that there is neither pressure gradient nor blood flow in the anastomoses of the circle of Willis connecting these arteries. It is interesting to note that blood from the vertebral arteries also supplies only the ipsilateral hemisphere, despite the fact that it passes along the common basilar artery. Direct observations on this vessel have shown that the flow of blood in its lumen is strictly laminar, as a result of which, if dye is injected into one of the vertebral arteries, it spreads only in the corresponding half of the lumen of the vessel and flows from it only into the ipsilateral arterial branches [202, 115].

Under normal conditions the system of the major arteries of the brain may provide a sufficient collateral blood supply to the brain after occlusion of a single internal carotid or vertebral artery. Cases frequently occur in clinical practice when occlusion of one, or even two of these arteries (atherosclerotic stenosis, thrombosis) is not reflected at all in the condition of the patients [154, 96, 70]. Similar results have been observed in experiments on animals [40, 103].

After occlusion of individual internal carotid arteries, the redistribution of blood into the other major arteries of the brain has been regarded by some workers as a purely passive hemodynamic phenomenon [347, 103]. However, experimental results suggest that following occlusion of one of the carotid arteries, the blood flow in the other is increased as a result of active responses of the major arteries of the brain in these processes. Many years ago, in his well known investigation, Rein [322, 323] showed that in dogs the blood flow in the common carotid artery could be doubled after occlusion of the contralateral vessel. This was not entirely because of elevation of the systemic arterial pressure, because these responses did not follow a

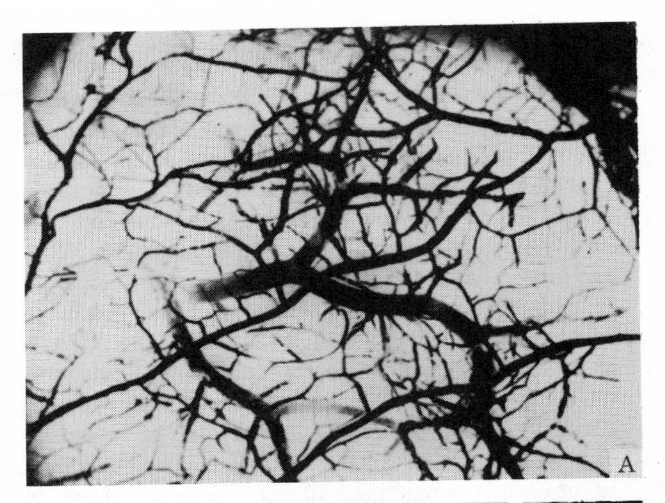

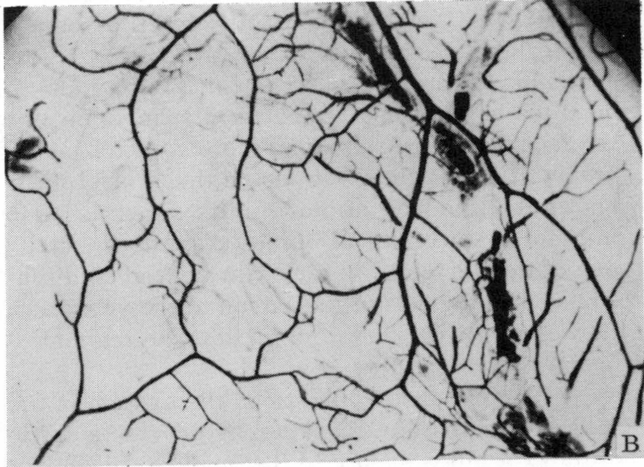

Fig. 41. Density of anastomotic arterial network on surface of cerebral hemispheres of different animals. Network of vessels injected with ink-gelatin mass. A) cat; B) rabbit (both, 16X). (Specimens prepared by L. G. Ormotsadze [223].)

completely parallel course (the increase in pressure always took place a little later). Dilatation of the system of the carotid artery evidently took place through a reflex from the carotid sinus, because after dissection of the vessels in that region to separate them from the surrounding tissues, no dilatation of the carotid arteries took place. This was later confirmed by other investigators [97, 241]. In some cases this compensation may be disturbed periodically, and then recover again: in clinical practice, neurological disturbances are frequently transient in character, with frequent and prolonged remissions [357]. The role of the circle of Willis as an anastomotic system supplying a collateral circulation has recently been studied by Himwich and co-workers [8, 44, 112] in experiments on animals, as well as on hydraulic, electrical, and mathematical models. The collateral blood supply to the brain after occlusion of one carotid artery is largely dependent on age changes in the vessel walls: whereas after occlusion of one internal carotid artery in young persons, the blood supply to the brain usually was not disturbed, in old people because of sclerosis of vessels of the circle of Willis, various neurological disturbances were frequently observed [354, 265]. An important role may also be played by the normal structure and functioning of the vessels of the circle of Willis. In a study of more than 1500 cadavers of persons with nervous and mental diseases, anomalies of its structure were found in 82% of cases [326]. Other workers who studied the anatomy of the circle of Willis found various forms of asymmetrical hypoplasia in 50% of cases [51],

The circle of Willis gives off the anterior, middle, and posterior cerebral arteries, which ramify successively to form a network of pial arteries that are distributed on the surface of the cerebral hemispheres, and are situated within comparatively large canals of the subarachnoid space [14]. The more highly developed the animal, the denser this network. In cats and dogs, for instance, it is much denser than in rabbits (Fig. 41). The presence of such a large number of anastomoses creates optimal conditions for a rapid collateral blood supply should one of the pial arteries become excluded. Those parts of the pial vascular system which possess the greatest number of anastomoses between branches of the middle cerebral artery, on the one hand, and branches of the anterior and posterior cerebral arteries on the other hand, have been called zones of mixed blood supply (Fig. 42) [160, 148].

Anastomoses of the pial arterial system, forming the anatomical basis of the collateral circulation, have been adequately studied [295, 148, 150, 391]. In particular, arteries which supply blood to phylogenetically older brain structures, such as the basal ganglia, have been shown to possess less well

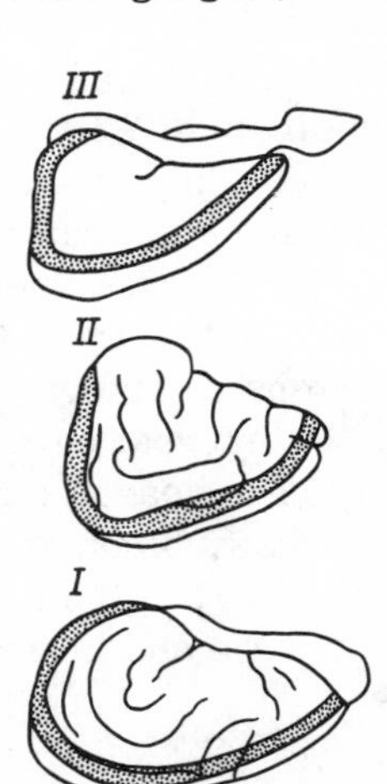

Fig. 42. Diagram showing position of zones of mixed blood supply of anterior, middle, and posterior cerebral arteries on lateral surface of cerebral hemispheres [148]. I) dog; II) cat; III) rabbit.

developed anastomoses, so that after their occlusion necrosis of the corresponding parts of the brain took place [168, 393]. On the other hand, the pial arteries on the brain surface, supplying blood to the cortex, constitute a rich anastomotic network, so that a collateral blood supply was more easily obtained after occlusion of their individual branches [137, 148, 376, 378]. Only if the radial arteries were occluded as they entered the cortex was the blood supply disturbed, for no arterial anastomoses are present within the brain substance, and the capillary network there could not maintain its blood supply [149, 87, 88].

An important factor for the collateral circulation in the brain is a normal level of the systemic arterial pressure. If this pressure is lowered, signs of inadequacy of the blood supply to the brain tissue develop. Experiments on animals in which the middle or anterior cerebral arteries were occluded showed that, if the systemic arterial pressure falls, signs of a deficient blood supply to the brain tissue appear immediately [159, 161, 149, 262]. Some workers have considered that an adequately high level of the arterial pressure is, indeed, the main factor essential for a collateral circulation in the brain following occlusion of individual intracranial arteries [161, 87, 88]. Clinical observations have shown that in patients with certain vascular diseases of the brain, such as atherosclerotic stenosis or thrombosis, neurological symptoms may not appear for a long time because of the collateral circulation. However, even a transient fall of the systemic arterial pressure is sufficient to cause the immediate appearance of signs of a deficient blood supply to the corresponding parts of the brain [46]. In experiments on monkeys, partial occlusion of the internal carotid arteries also was unaccompanied by the development of symptoms, but if the systemic arterial pressure fell, changes appeared in the electroencephalogram indicating a deficient blood supply to the cerebral cortex; these changes were reversible [47, 331]. This phenomenon is regarded as one type of "dynamic disturbance of the cerebral circulation" [188]. However, a sharp increase in the systemic arterial pressure can also prevent a collateral blood supply, because under these conditions a diffuse constriction of the pial arteries to 50% of their initial diameter was observed [271].

In view of the previous widely held opinion that the cerebral vessels are relatively passive and devoid of nervous control, no attention has been paid to their active role in the collateral circulation. Usually attention has been concentrated on anatomical factors (the existence of anastomoses and the absence of sclerotic changes in the vessel walls), and also on a factor acting mechanically on the collateral circulation (a normal level of the systemic arterial pressure [161, 87, 88, 262], leaving open the question of the role of the active functional behavior of arteries of the brain itself in the development of the collateral circulation. It was not until after 1960 that the functional behavior of the brain vessels after occlusion of the individual pial arteries in rabbits was studied by the author [239, 240, 255]. The responses of the vascular network peripheral to the site of occlusion was studied by serial photomicrography and subsequent measurement of the diameter of the vessels on photographic film by means of an occular micrometer. After occlusion by galvanic or diathermy current of a relatively large pial artery, 80-100 μ in diameter (usually a branch of the middle cerebral artery), dilatation of its peripheral portion, and of all its branches and anastomoses took place, the dilatation being greater in the case of small arteries than of large (Fig. 43). Dilatation began immediately after occlusion, reached its maximum during the first minute, and most branches then gradually narrowed again to their initial diameter, only a few pial arteries remaining dilated. The initial generalized dilatation of the vessels in rabbits is evidently a manifestation of "overregulation" (i.e., an excessively strong regulatory response), and later only those arteries providing a collateral blood supply to the bed of the occluded vessel stay dilated [239, 240]. In similar experiments on cats, vasodilatation of the pial arteries in these animals did not develop at once peripherally to the point of occlusion; only the smaller anastomoses through which the collateral blood supply must

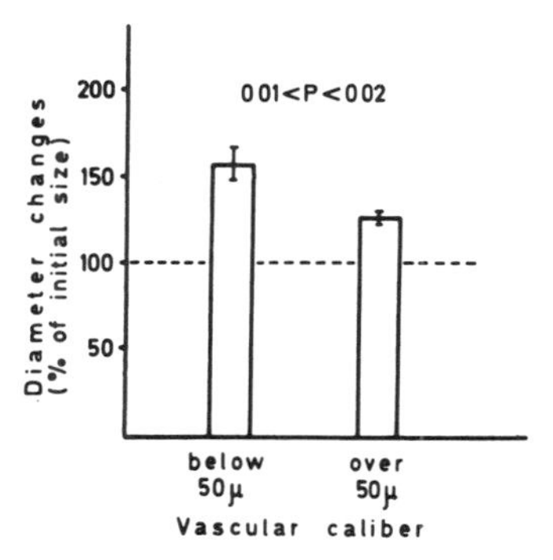

Fig. 43. The degree of dilatation of pial arteries peripheral to the site of occlusion, in percent of their initial diameter (100%) depending on whether diameter is under or over 50 μ [240] (arithmetic means and standard deviations).

be obtained undergo dilatation [89]. Later work on rabbits show that the dilator response of the pial arteries occurred only peripherally to the occluded segment, and the portion of the artery located proximally (i.e., nearer the heart) was usually constricted [240]. The length of the constricted segment did not exceed 1 mm, but the degree of constriction was sometimes very considerable, amounting in some cases to the complete closure to the lumen of the vessel (in an undamaged part of the artery). This vasoconstriction seems to be of the same origin as that in the area of vascular damage.

Peripheral to the site of occlusion, concurrent with dilatation of the pial arteries, some branches of arteries could be seen which had not hitherto been visible under the microscope [239, 240]. These were anastomoses between branches of the occluded vessel and neighboring pial arteries. Measurements made on the photographic film after photomicrography of the brain surface of rabbits showed that the diameter of the anastomoses when they began to function did not exceed 45 μ. The responses of the arterial anastomoses in the zone of mixed blood supply of the middle, anterior, and posterior cerebral arteries were studied next in total microscopic preparations of the pia fixed intravitally *in situ* from the surface (using 20% formalin solution in alcohol). In one group of rabbits all large branches of the middle cerebral arteries were occluded, while in others (controls), the pial arteries remained intact. In none of these groups of rabbits were the arterial anastomoses as a rule completely closed. However, some of them did not participate in the circulation, because they were filled with plasma only, and not with erythrocytes (Fig. 44). Measurement of the diameter of the anastomoses in these specimens showed that after occlusion of the middle cerebral artery it increased on the average from 22 ± 1 to 28 ± 1.5 μ ($P < 0.001$); at the same time, considerably fewer of the plasma-filled vessels were found: 40 ± 7.1% compared with 85 ± 6.4% in the control animals ($P < 0.001$). Some anastomoses contained few erythrocytes and were intermediate forms between inactive and active arterial anastomoses. The hemodynamic mechanisms of origin of the plasma-filled vessels and their role in changes in the local circulation were studied by the author in other organs previously [208]. Hence, whereas injection of contrast materials into the cerebral vessels in previous investigations [137, 148, 391] revealed the anatomy of arterial anastomoses on the brain surface, the later investigations now described revealed some of their functional characteristics.

Radial arteries branch from the pial arteries roughly at right angles to the brain surface, pene-

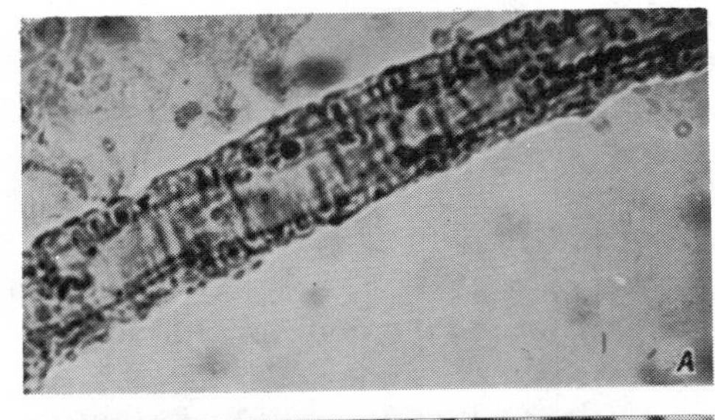

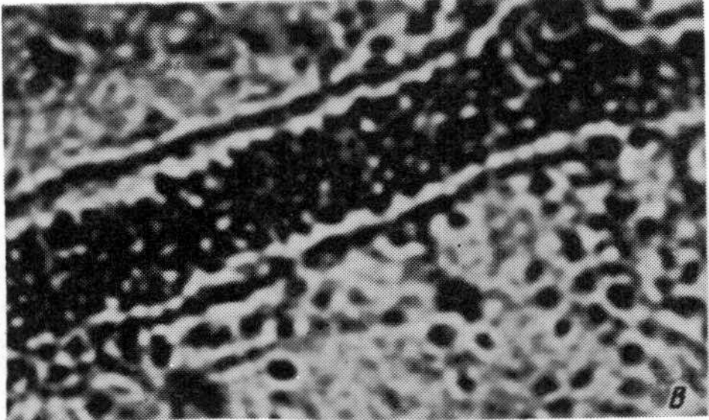

Fig. 44. Different functional states of the arterial anastomoses in a zone of mixed blood supply of the middle, anterior, and posterior cerebral arteries of the rabbit. A) nonfunctioning anastomosis filled only with blood plasma; B) one of the anastomoses becoming active after occlusion of branches of middle cerebral artery. Photomicrographs of total preparations of pia mater fixed intravitally from brain surface, 56X [240].

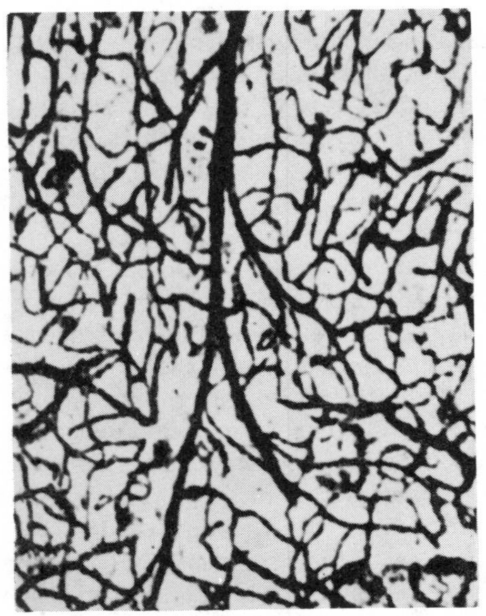

Fig. 45. Ramification of radial artery in anterior sylvian gyrus of a puppy. Vascular network impregnated with silver by Klosovskii's method. Photomicrograph, 10X [148].

trate into the brain tissue, and ramify to form a capillary plexus (Fig. 45). Unlike the larger arteries – the major trunks and the pial arteries – the intracerebral arteries are not connected by anastomoses [148]. The capillary plexus is continuous throughout the brain tissues. Its density varies considerably in different parts of the brain. It has been found that the more numerous the mitochondria in the tissue elements of a particular part of the brain, i.e., the greater the intensity of its metabolism, the richer the capillary plexus [339]. The network of vessels is much denser in the gray matter than in the white [186]. The structure of the capillary plexus is so specific in different parts of the brain, and even in different layers of the cortex, that some decades ago it provided the foundations for a theory of cerebral angioarchitectonics [308]. Capillary networks in the cerebral cortex of various species of animals have been studied in recent years [183, 184, 185]. The capillaries are the only link between the arteries and veins of the brains, because arteriovenous anastomoses are not found in the brain, unlike in most other organs [148, 330].

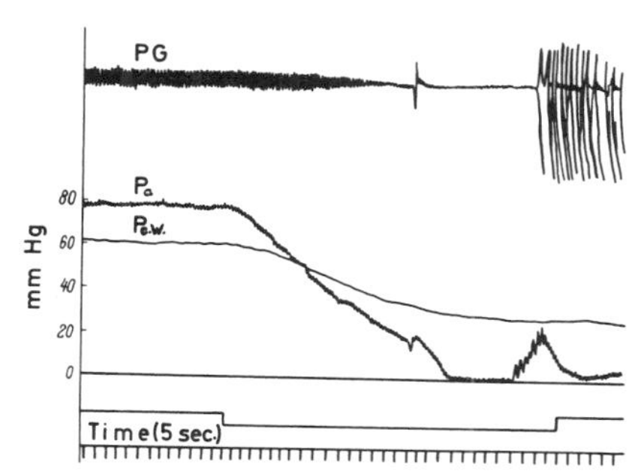

Fig. 46. Phenomenon of crossing of pressures in a rabbit in the terminal state [213]. PG, tracing of respiration; P_a, systemic arterial pressure; $P_{c.W.}$, pressure in circle of Willis. Marker shows period of bleeding from abdominal aorta.

Terminal State Preceding Death

The functional behavior of the brain vessels becomes very active if the systemic arterial pressure falls to zero (or almost to zero), as, for instance, in terminal states [213] or during temporary occlusion of the aorta [231]. In experiments on rabbits, regardless of the cause of death (cardiac arrest following injection of ether into the myocardium, bleeding from the abdominal aorta, or asphyxia through closure of the trachea), the following phenomenon was found: during a comparatively rapid fall of systemic arterial pressure, the pressure in a manometer connected via the internal carotid artery to the circle of Willis fell much more slowly (Figs. 31 and 46) [213]. This phenomenon was observed in 85% of the author's experiments (26 animals), and the curves showing these pressures crosses at different levels, from 20 to 70 mm Hg. This effect could arise through the following causes. First, the pressure in the circle of Willis is in fact higher than in the aorta, for dissociation of the two systems of vessels takes place through sharp constriction of the internal carotid and vertebral arteries [213]; otherwise, when the aortic pressure

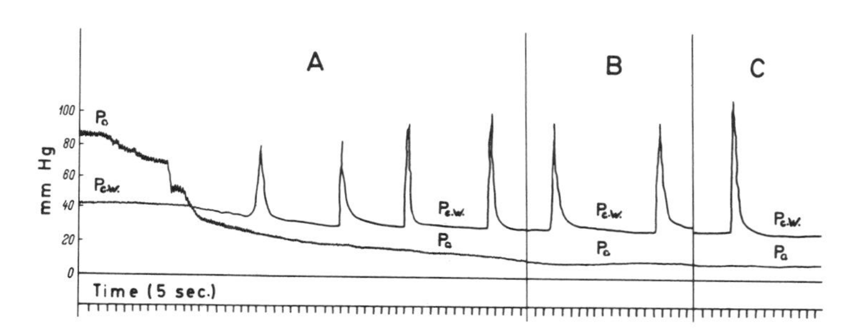

Fig. 47. The "critical closing pressure" of internal carotid artery after development of terminal state in a rabbit [215]. P_a, systemic arterial pressure; $P_{c.W.}$, pressure in circle of Willis. B) 6 min, and C) 18 min after crossing of pressure curves on trace A. During artificial elevation of pressure in manometer measuring pressure in circle of Willis, it falls rapidly, but at a certain level (from 30-40 mm Hg) it ceases to fall through closure of the artery. Level of venous pressure in transverse sinus 8 (B) and 7 (C) mm Hg.

fell, a rapid retrograde flow of blood would take place from the circle of Willis along the wide major arteries of the brain into the aorta until the pressures in them were equalized. Second, marked constriction of the internal carotid artery connecting the circle of Willis with the manometer takes place; the readings of the manometer therefore reflect the fall in pressure in the circle of Willis with relatively high inertia. The phenomenon described above thus indicates sharp constriction of the major arteries of the brain if the aortic pressure falls to (or almost to) zero. In some experiments on rabbits, the internal carotid artery connecting the circle of Willis with the manometer was constricted until its lumen was completely closed, so that the "critical closing pressure" of this vessel could be recorded [215]. It will be clear from Fig. 47, that after injection of fluid into the manometer system connected with the internal carotid artery, the pressure in it rises, but it immediately starts to fall because the fluid passes through this artery to enter the vascular system of the brain; however, as soon as the pressure reaches a certain level, it ceases to fall, evidently because of complete closure of the lumen of the internal carotid artery. This same phenomenon could be observed many times over if the test was repeated. In these experiments a critical closing pressure of this artery is thus found, at which its level remains about the same for many minutes, or falls gradually. In the experiment described above it was 30-40 mm Hg, whereas in the venous sinuses of the brain the pressure did not exceed 10 mm Hg. The presence of a critical closing pressure indicates that the sharp constriction of the major arteries of the brain discovered in terminal states is not the result of thrombosis of the vessels, but of their vasoconstriction, i.e., it is a manifestation of the functional behavior of the vessel wall. This same phenomenon apparently was observed previously in rabbits [40]: during a fall of the systemic arterial pressure, at the level of about 30 mm Hg the total cerebrovascular resistance (from the arteries to the veins of the brain) rose suddenly and sharply; at that time, the authors cited did not know which vessels are constricted but now, on the basis of the experiments described above, it is evident that it was the major arteries of the brain.

The phenomenon described above, concerning the relatively high pressure in a manometer connected to the circle of Willis, is observed during the terminal state in dogs also (Fig. 48) although to a much less marked degree, possibly because of the existence of extensive anastomoses between the internal carotid arteries and branches of the maxillary arteries. In fatal cases of embolism, it has also been observed [50] that the pressure in the circle of Willis can remain for some time at a relatively high level, whereas the systemic arterial pressure falls to zero. A slow decrease of pressure in the circle of Willis has also been described after severe blood loss in animals [164]. Sharp constriction of the internal carotid arteries of dogs in response to lowering of the systemic arterial pressure during terminal states is also indicated

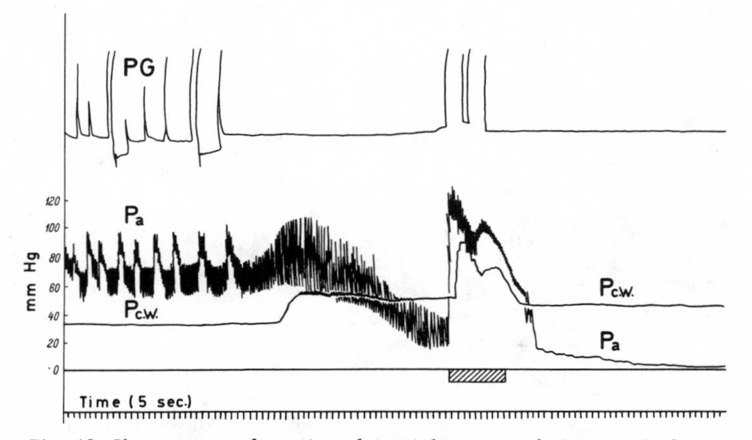

Fig. 48. Phenomenon of crossing of arterial pressures during terminal state in a dog (experiments by G. I. Mchedlishvili and L. G. Ormotsadze [223]. PG, respiration; P_a, systemic arterial pressure; $P_{c.w.}$, pressure in circle of Willis. Temporary artificial increase of systemic arterial pressure by means of compensator (marker under zero line) does not change the course of the curves.

by the results of experiments in which the blood flow was measured (by means of a flowmeter) and in which the resistance in these vessels was determined [180, 181].

Morphological investigations [73] have also shown that constriction of a particular segment of the internal carotid arteries may develop during a sudden fall in the systemic arterial pressure; one of the illustrations to this paper shows a distinctive change in shape and narrowing of this artery. To avoid possible postmortem changes in the vessels, in later investigations by the present author [210] the walls of the internal carotid and vertebral arteries of rabbits and dogs were fixed intravitally by injection of 20% formalin in alcohol shortly before death. A study of serial microscopic sections and corrosion specimens showed that these arteries are not constricted throughout their length, but only in certain areas, approximately in the same situation in both rabbits and dogs: for the internal carotid arteries, mainly in the carotid canal in the pyramid of the temporal bone and in the cavernous sinus, and for the vertebral arteries, in the region of the flexures of these vessels and of their entry to the subarachnoid spaces of the brain.

The marked constriction of the internal carotid and also, evidently, the vertebral arteries during a fall of systemic arterial pressure almost to zero has thus been demonstrated by different methods. This constriction evidently takes place when the systemic arterial pressure is about 30 mm Hg, although the methods so far used have not enabled this level to be established exactly. The physiological importance of this phenomenon is not yet clear. We can only postulate that in the case of complete closure of the lumen of the major arteries to the brain, blood is unable to flow in the retrograde direction from the circle of Willis into the aorta, and the blood pressure in the arteries of the brain cannot therefore fall as quickly as the systemic arterial pressure. The pressure gradient in the vascular system of the brain is still maintained for the time being, and may enable a weak flow of arterial blood to continue in the cerebral capillaries [213]. Naturally, the higher the blood pressure remains in the circle of Willis, the better the animal can tolerate a decrease in systemic arterial pressure; in experiments in which animals were bled repeatedly (every 40-60 min), the writer showed that the pressure in the circle of Willis could be maintained at successively higher levels (for example, 10, 14, 30, and 52 mm Hg), and in all possibility this helped the animal to withstand repeated terminal states [214].

The distinctive behavior of the pial arteries of rabbits in terminal states has been revealed by serial photomicrography. In the initial period of a fall in systemic arterial pressure (Figs. 49 and 30), all the pial arteries are slightly dilated (probably a reaction to reduction of the pressure, e.g., above, p. 23). However, starting from the time of constriction of the major arteries of the brain (where the pressure curves cross each other) the larger pial arteries begin to dilate and the smaller to constrict; later the former begin to constrict and the latter to dilate (blood is thereby switched from the larger into the smaller pial arteries). These successive dilatations and constrictions of the pial arteries can be repeated [213]. Similar phenomena have been found after occlusion of the aorta in dogs, when the larger pial arteries (of the order of 300 μ) began to constrict gradually, while the smaller arteries (about 50 μ) began to dilate [231]. The general impression is obtained that a slow peristaltic wave moves along the pial arteries in the orthograde directions. Since the cerebral cortex receives its blood supply through the pial vessels, it could be concluded that the blood flow also continues in its capillaries. In rabbits, a circulation in

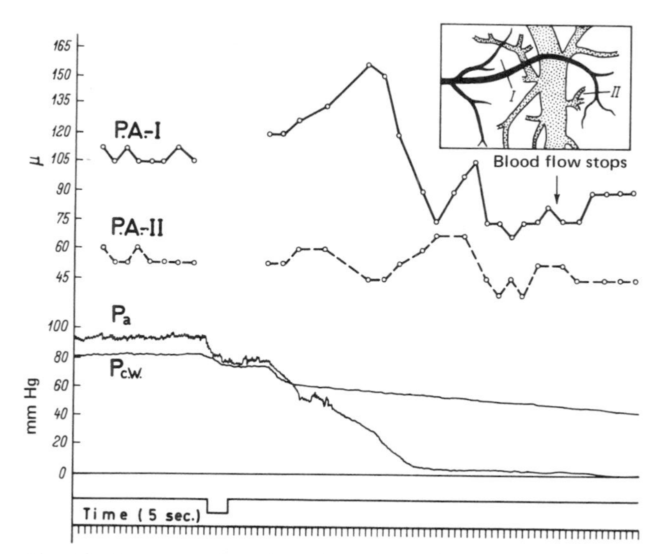

Fig. 49. Changes in functional behavior of the pial arteries, characteristic of a terminal state, in a rabbit. They resemble a wave of peristaltic contraction of the vessel walls and are evidently responsible for continuation of the orthograde blood flow in the cerebral vessels (stopping of the blood flow marked by an arrow on the figure) [213]. P.A.(I), diameter of large, and P.A.(II), of small pial arteries (these vessels are shown schematically in the diagram in the top right-hand corner, taken from a photomicrograph); P_a, systemic arterial pressure; $P_{c.W.}$, blood pressure in circle of Willis. Marker shows time of injection of ether into myocardium.

the pial vessels was observed for about as long as the "peristalsis" of the arteries continued, i.e., for 2-3 min [213]. In dogs, after occlusion of the aorta and temporary stoppage of the blood flow in the pial vessels, it sometimes started again, gradually quickening and reaching a maximum, and then starting to slow once again; after 4-6 min it stopped completely. If the lumen of the aorta remained closed, the restoration of the blood flow in the pial vessels was not repeated, because the compensatory powers of the animal were evidently exhausted and death ensued [231].

The existence of this phenomenon was confirmed by investigations using other methods. Measurements of the blood flow in the cortex in cats with Gibbs' needles showed [181, 182] that circulatory arrest takes place after the systemic arterial pressure falls; so far as the oxygen tension measured polarographically in the brain is concerned, in some cases this even increased, while in others its decrease was delayed, and finally, in some experiments it fell rapidly (evidently if compensation was poor). Another investigation showed [165] that the oxygen tension in the cortex and subcortex of dogs falls more slowly than the blood pressure in the aorta and in the circle of Willis.

The presence of this reduced circulation of blood in the brain may perhaps influence the length of survival of its neurons after the systemic arterial pressure falls. To test this hypothesis, it was necessary to compare the "survival time" (the time taken for spontaneous cortical electrical activity to disappear after cessation of the blood supply to the brain) in animals of the same species in the presence and absence of this reduced circulation in the brain. In experiments in which the blood flow to the brain was arrested by application of an inflatable cuff to the animal's neck or by stopping perfusion of the isolated head, it was still possible for this reduced circulation to take place; the mean survival time of the rabbits in these experiments was 20-25 sec [113]. In experiments undertaken jointly by the writer with A. I. Roitbak [223] the conditions were such that the blood flow in the cerebral capillaries must have stopped instantaneously. A suspension of lycopodium was injected rapidly into an artery of the brain; its particles, 30-40 μ in diameter, block the smallest pial and intracerebral arterioles, and it was found that the reduced circulation in the cerebral capillaries could not be maintained despite the operation of the vascular mechanisms of the brain described above. Spontaneous electrical activity in the rabbit's cortex stopped after 5-10 sec, and paroxysmal discharges produced by local application of strychnine to the cortex disappeared after 2-3 sec (Fig. 50). This indicates that, when the mechanism responsible for the reduced circulation in the brain in terminal states are excluded, the survival time of the cortical neurons is considerably shorter.

However, this weak motion of arterial blood in the cerebral capillaries under these conditions could be, of course, insufficient to provide for even the minimal metabolic requirements of the brain, more especially because the low intracapillary pressure must prevent the passage of substances from the blood into the brain tissue. Attention must therefore be directed to the unique behavior of the

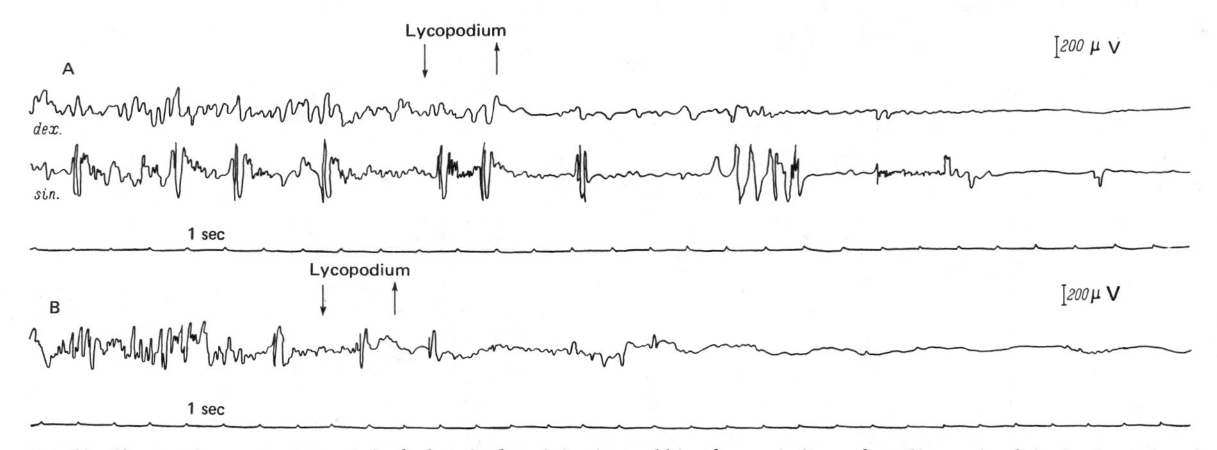

Fig. 50. Changes in spontaneous cortical electrical activity in a rabbit after embolism of small vessels of the brain produced by lycopodium particles (marked by arrows) in two experiments (A and B). Trace A shows paroxysmal discharges in the left hemisphere (sin.) after local application of strychnine. (Experiments of G. I. Mchedlishvili and A. I. Roitbak [223].) Explanation in text.

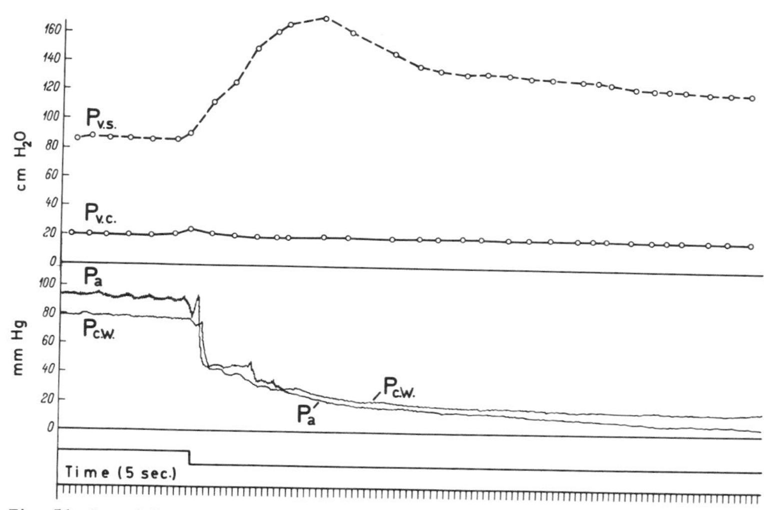

Fig. 51. Local increase in venous pressure in sinuses of the brain during terminal state in a rabbit. The increased pressure gradient thus produced along the course of the emissary veins of the skull indicates their constriction [213]. $P_{v.s.}$, venous pressure in transverse sinus; $P_{v.c.}$, pressure in cranial (superior) vena cava; P_a, systemic arterial pressure; $P_{c.W.}$, pressure in circle of Willis. Marker shows time of injection of ether into myocardium.

venous system of the brain, which seems to prevent the blood pressure in its capillaries from falling when the systemic arterial pressure is lowered [213, 231]. Experiments showed that even when the pressure in the circle of Willis was low, the venous pressure in the sinuses of the brain was raised, although the pressure in the large veins of the thorax remained unchanged or was increased to a lesser degree (Fig. 51). These results showed that the increase in venous pressure in the brain was local and, in all probability, the result of the reduced outflow of blood via the emissary veins of the skull. Judging from the pressure gradient, the resistance in these veins was increased by several times, although it is not yet known which segments of the emissary veins undergo constriction. When the systemic arterial pressure falls sharply, the conditions thereby created naturally in the brain are thus similar to those produced artificially in a limb with a disturbed blood supply (because of endarteritis, etc.), when the surgeon attempts to obtain some improvement in tissue nutrition by ligating the venous trunks [297].

The presence of mechanisms maintaining a weak blood flow and blood pressure in the capillaries when the systemic arterial pressure falls is evidently characteristic of the brain because nothing like it has yet been found in other parts of the body. Although the blood flow produced in this way in the capillaries is very weak, it may be of some importance in keeping the brain alive, because it has been shown that as little as 10% of the normal circulation in the brain is adequate for that purpose [344].

The functional behavior of the vascular mechanisms of the brain described above is evidently the reason why it is possible to resuscitate an animal or man, when in a state of agony or clinical death, by means of intra-arterial blood transfusion in conjunction with other measures. However, in the course of the present author's investigation of the cerebral circulation in terminal states it was found that the compensatory mechanisms of the arterial and venous systems of the brain, as described above, function by no means equally well in every animal. Although no special study has yet been undertaken to determine under what conditions this happens, it can be assumed that disturbance of the function of the compensatory mechanisms depends on the depth of anesthesia, and on the physiological state and age of the organism. If attempts are made to resuscitate an animal or man in the presence of such disturbances, it is certain either that they will fail or that they will be followed by complications in the form of postischemic brain lesions, including edema and various neurological disorders.

CHAPTER IV

CAUSES OF PRIMARY DISTURBANCE OF THE CEREBRAL CIRCULATION

There may be several different causes of disturbance of the cerebral circulation. In conformity with the general plan of this book, in this chapter we shall examine only those disorders of blood flow in the brain which are produced by primary disturbances of the normal functional behavior of the vascular mechanisms of the brain, and we shall not consider circulatory disturbances of the type that are caused by sclerotic changes in the cerebral vessels or by their thrombosis and embolism. In general, functional disturbances of the cerebral circulation can depend, on the one hand, on extrinsic causes: significant changes in the level of the systemic arterial and venous pressures and, consequently, changes in the inflow of blood into the brain or its outflow from the skull. On the other hand, they can be due to intrinsic causes: a local increase of resistance in the vessels of the brain itself. In each of these causes, compensatory mechanisms belonging to the cerebral circulation begin to function, and within certain limits they diminish or even abolish completely the circulatory disturbances arising in the brain. Although disturbances of the cerebral circulation are well compensated in the body, the results of activity of the compensatory mechanisms of the cerebral circulation are effective, from the point of view of abolishing the ensuing disorders, in by no means every case: they may not function equally well in different organisms (in animals of the same species and, in particular, in animals at different levels of phylogenetic development); even within the same organism, compensatory mechanisms may not always function equally effectively depending on the concrete conditions in force at the time; their function may also have its negative aspect, i.e., by compensating one disturbance they may give rise to other circulatory disturbances or may contribute to their production.

Bearing in mind that the functioning of compensatory mechanism of the cerebrovascular system under several conditions has been fully examined in the previous chapters, we shall examine below only those functional changes in the cerebrovascular system which can give rise to disorders of the blood supply to the brain, i.e., which are purely pathological changes.

Spasm of the Cerebral Arteries

By contrast with physiological vasoconstriction, spasm describes a purely pathological constriction of arteries which a) is characterized by considerable magnitude and duration, b) is an unrelaxing contraction of the muscular coat of the vessel, c) is not related to the needs of the organism under the particular conditions concerned (i.e., is not compensatory), and d) leads to a sharp decrease in the blood flow in the affected vessel, so that in the absence of a collateral inflow of blood, it disturbs the blood supply of the corresponding organ.

Doubts were expressed for a long time whether spasm of the cerebral vessels can occur, in fact almost until the 1960's, although clinicians had always found it easiest to explain some types of disturbances in the brain by functional spasm of the cerebral arteries. These doubts were based, first, on the impossibility of proving the existence of spasm at that time in patients because of the lack of adequate methods of investigation and second, on the fact that in autopsy material spasm had never been demonstrated histopathologically in any vessels of the brain. For these reasons, the problem of spasm of the cerebral arteries had first to be studied experimentally in animals. Only then, by extrapolation to man and by special investigation on patients, could the problem be resolved under clinical conditions.

The possible localization of spasm of the cerebral arteries can be determined only if the functional properties of different parts of the arterial system of the brain are known. Without such knowledge, many investigators worked simply by a method of trial and error, and attempted to produce spasm experimentally in a number of different arteries in the brain. Since the pial arteries are the most easily accessible for investigation, many workers attempted to study spasm of these arteries on the brain surface. Powerful constriction of the pial arteries, resembling spasm, has been observed in animal experiments in response to direct mechanical or electrical stimulation of their walls. The first observations were made about 100 years ago [348], when sharp constriction of the pial arteries was observed in response to direct electrical stimulation. This phenomenon was later studied in more detail by other workers. During mechanical stimulation of the walls of the pial arteries, a sharp local constriction took place, amounting in some cases to complete closure of the lumen of the vessel, lasting for between a few seconds and 10 minutes or more (in cats and rabbits) [74]. In the case of electrical stimulation, the stronger the stimulus the stronger and more prolonged the contraction of the arterial walls. Some arteries were refractory to stimulation from the very beginning, while others became refractory after the vessel wall had been stimulated and had contracted into a state of spasm. These results were confirmed in general by later experiments on cats, dogs, and monkeys, but in general it was more difficult to produce spasm in monkeys than in dogs, and more difficult still than in cats [61]. The sensitivity of the pial arteries to mechanical and, in particular, to electrical stimulation and their ability to contract in a manner resembling spasm differed not only among different arteries, but also in the same vessels in the course of the experiment: usually their sensitivity gradually diminished and then began to recover again. Later experiments [342] showed that spasm of the pial arteries may also take place in response to mechanical stimulation of their walls from within, such as during obstruction with glass wool (rats, rabbits, cats, and dogs).

Tests with a variety of substances applied directly to the pial arteries of cats, dogs, and monkeys showed that by far the great majority of them had no effect either by producing or abolishing the spasm of the pial arteries. Local application of serotonin to the vascular walls caused only an insignificant and short constriction of the pial arteries in cats [319], and failed to produce spasm of the middle cerebral artery in monkeys [377]. A weak and inconstant effect of this substance on the pial arteries has been observed also in rabbits [300]. The same results were obtained with catecholamines [377]. However it has been reported that the adrenolytic drug phentolamine decreased spasm of the pial arteries caused by direct electrical stimulation of the vascular walls [177]. Marked constriction of the pial arteries was observed after local application of 5% barium chloride [330] and, in the author's experiments, of hypotonic saline to the pial arterial walls, when the width of the vessels was reduced by up to 30% of its initial value. However, the constriction was short in duration, reaching a maximum in 10-15 sec and then gradually disappearing (after about 1 min).

Among natural conditions which have been observed to cause a strong and prolonged constriction of the pial arteries similar to vasospasm, experimental renal hypertension may be mentioned; in this condition the systemic arterial pressure reached 200 mm Hg [39]. An important role in this case must have been played by hypertensive substances circulating in the blood stream, for the same elevation of the arterial pressure, if produced mechanically (by compression of the thoracic aorta below arteries supplying the brain), gave rise not to typical spasm, but to only a partial constriction (not more than 50%) of the whole system of pial arteries [271].

These considerations suggest that, though the pial arteries are able to constrict as in vascular spasm in response to artificial stimulation of the blood vessel walls, under natural conditions spasm of single pial arteries of experimental animals has never been regularly obtained. It can thus be considered either that the pial arteries are not a typical locus of spasm in the cerebral vascular system or that the workers cited were unaware of those preliminary changes in the vessel walls which were necessary for the appearance of typical spasm after natural vasoconstrictor stimulation of the pial arterial walls.

Pathological constriction, resembling spasm, of the major arteries of the brain has been observed clinically and in experimental animals since the late 1950s, i.e., about simultaneously with the discovery of their active responses and their important role in the regulation of the blood supply to the brain. Following injection of x-ray contrast material, marked constriction of the internal carotid arteries has been found in man [37]. It has also been revealed by angiography in patients with clinical evidence of a disturbance of the blood supply to the brain [315, 178, 133] and also during migraine attacks [59]. In the course of surgical operations in which the bony canal through which the internal carotid artery passes was opened,

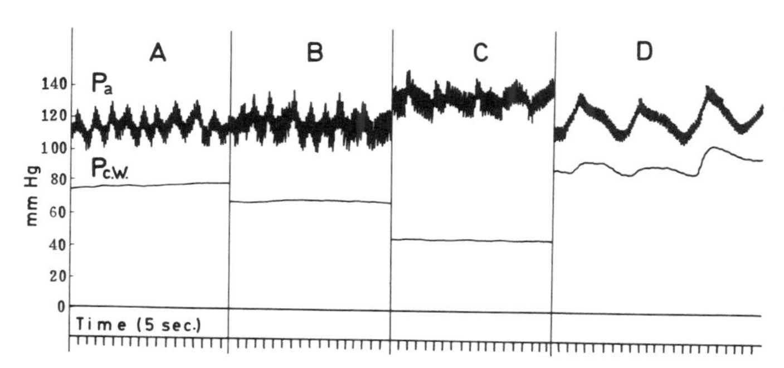

Fig. 52. Changes in pressure gradient in the system of major arteries of the brain in a dog during the development of spasm (A, B, C) and after its removal (D) [221]. P_a, systemic arterial pressure; $P_{c.W.}$, pressure in circle of Willis; A) original state; B) 30 min later; C) another 12 min later; D) another 50 min later.

it was noted [313] that, in response to mechanical stimulation, the walls of this vessel contract sharply as if in spasm. Constriction of the spasm type has recently been observed in the carotid system by the use of a special modification of rheoencephalography during an investigation of mental fatigue in schoolchildren [317, 368] and also by other methods in patients with various cerebrovascular disorders [84].

In animal experiments typical spasm of the major arteries of the brain was demonstrated by the author in the early 1960s. Initial simultaneous constriction of the whole system of these arteries, leading to a decrease in the blood supply to the brain, was observed [221]. In these experiments the resistance in the major arteries rose, apparently spontaneously, during the acute stage, while the pressure in the aorta remained unchanged, and that in the circle of Willis fell progressively. Evidence of cerebral ischemia was given by typical changes in the electrocorticogram of the animals, i.e., by the appearance of slow waves and a marked decrease in amplitude of the EEG. This angiospasm usually developed gradually, over a period ranging from a few hours in some cases to 15-30 min in others (Fig. 52); less often constriction of these arteries occurred almost instantaneously (Fig. 53).

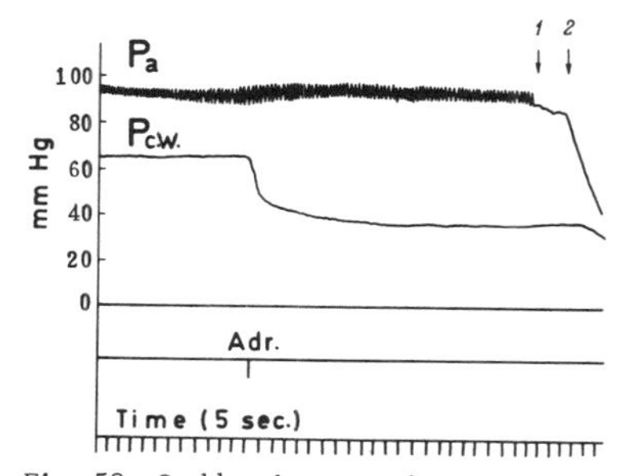

Fig. 53. Sudden increase in resistance resulting from development of spasm in the system of major arteries of the brain in a rabbit following intra-aortic injection of adrenalin (100 μg). Experiment on thorax-head preparation [321]. P_a, intra-aortic pressure; $P_{c.W.}$, pressure in circle of Willis. Marker shows time of injection of the drug. Spasm of major arteries of brain caused a fall of blood pressure in the circle of Willis; cardiac arrest (1) and death (2) quickly ensued.

If the spasm of the brain arteries did not disappear, the animal died, and the prognosis regarding the period of survival of the experimental animal could be made on the basis of the rate of development of spasm of these arteries. In cats, in which the internal carotid artery is almost obliterated, its function can be taken over by the rete mirabile connecting the branches of the external carotid artery with the circle of Willis. The present author, in a joint investigation with Dr. D. Ingvar,* observed that with the spontaneous development of functional constriction of these blood vessels the intensity of the circulation in the parietal cortex was reduced on the average by half (quantitative determination using the radioactive krypton clearance method [123]); about 30 min later the intensity of the circulation was restored to its initial level through the collateral inflow of blood from the contralateral carotid system.

Constriction of the major arteries of the brain resembling spasm has also been observed by other

*These experiments were carried out in 1963 in the Department of Clinical Neurophysiology of the University of Lund, Sweden.

investigators in animal experiments under various conditions. In cats, for instance, constriction of the walls of the intracranial portion of the internal carotid artery in response to direct mechanical stimulation of the vessel in control experiments lasted 1.5–8.5 min, while after injection of radioopaque material into the common carotid artery toward the brain, it lasted from 2 to 5 times longer [320]. In addition, 24 h after exposure of rabbits to ionizing radiation, a series of changes in the cerebral circulation was discovered; in particular, a much higher pressure had to be used to inject the radioopaque material for angiography [191]. The author cited considers perfectly justifiably that this was the result of constriction in the region of the "closing mechanisms" of the major arteries of brain. In another investigation [284] to study the direct responses of the vascular system in rabbits to irradiation, the blood pressure in the circle of Willis fell considerably in cases when the systemic arterial pressure was unchanged. The larger the dose of irradiation, the greater the increase in resistance in the major arteries, which indicated that constriction of this arterial system took place. During a prolonged fall of arterial pressure in dogs with traumatic shock, the sooner the blood pressure in the circle of Willis began to fall, the more rapidly agony developed [392], thus indicating the great importance of development of spasm of the major arteries of the brain in this case. Similar constriction of the system of major arteries of the brain, which developed gradually, also was observed during posthemorrhagic arterial hypotension in rabbits and dogs [3].

The genesis of pathological constriction of the major arteries of the brain is a problem of particular interest. It was observed by the author [221] very early in the investigations that spasm of the major arteries of the brain develops in cases when factors leading to a comparatively brief constriction of these arteries are repeated frequently (elevation of the pressure in most venous sinuses of the brain, terminal states, complete occlusion of the aorta or of the cranial vena cava, a marked increase in intracranial pressure, and so on). Apparently in response to repeated vasoconstrictor influences on the system of the internal carotid and vertebral arteries, they ultimately may go into prolonged and persistent constriction resembling spasm

The present author has undertaken further experimental investigations of the genesis of spasm of the internal carotid arteries using improved methods: initially by measuring the blood flow in the artery and finally by two modifications of resistography of the isolated internal carotid artery *in situ* in dogs (see Chapter I). It was noted that the tendency for spasm of the internal carotid arteries to develop was particularly marked in old animals, in experiments when the incidence of its development was much higher. Further investigations showed that for spasm of the major arteries of the brain to develop, conditions must be provided under which, in response to vasoconstrictor stimuli (local application of exogenous vasoconstrictor substances, reflex vasoconstrictor effects, elevation of the intravascular pressure, and so on) the vessel wall contracts, but for some reason or other its subsequent relaxation is disturbed. Experiments on the internal carotid artery isolated *in situ* showed that during spasm the resistance in the vessel may increase to such an extent that the blood flow (or even the flow of Ringer's solution, despite its low viscosity) becomes impossible even when the perfusion pressure is raised to 300-350 mm Hg.

Tests on the internal carotid artery of dogs, isolated *in situ*, showed [245] that even if spasm of this artery during the experiment was complete and unrelaxing, after the animal died, and the artery was dissected and fixed in formalin, no spasm could be found. These experiments thus showed that the typical arterial spasm existing during life disappears after death, and it was clear why pathologists had never been able to observe spasm of the cerebral arteries in the cadaver, even if present before death. The author of this book was able to observe the internal carotid artery of dogs in a state of spasm only with the aid of special conditions.

The method used for this purpose was based on the fact that an increase in the potassium ion concentration in the perfusion fluid (at the expense of sodium) leads to a sharp, but easily reversible (after restoration of the normal K^+ concentration) spasm of the internal carotid artery in dogs. Accordingly, in order to investigate spasm of these arteries morphologically, they were injected intravitally under constant pressure (100-120 mm Hg) with Ringer's solution in which the K^+ concentration was increased by about 5-8 times, oxygenated and warmed to 37°C. The animal was quickly sacrificed (either by exsanguination from the femoral artery or by injection of 10-15 ml ether into the heart), but perfusion of the internal carotid artery was continued during death of the vascular wall: for the first 3-4 h at 37°C and thereafter at room temperature. The perfusion fluid was then changed to 10% neutral formalin, made up in the same Ringer's solution, and perfusion of the vessel continued until next day. The artery was thus fixed in the state of spasm, and this allowed corrosion specimens of the vessel to be made and the vessel wall to be investigated histologically.

Investigation of internal carotid arteries fixed in a state of spasm, and also of the outlines of their lumen on corrosion specimens under the binocular microscope showed [245] that the artery was constricted throughout its length and, in particular, in the region of its flexure, where frequently the lumen was reduced by 67-80% compared with the control. The constriction was usually irregular, and frequently the configuration of the vessel was altered: complex twistings and invaginations of the wall, etc., appeared. Since the loss of pressure in a vessel in general is proportional to the fourth power of its radius, it could be concluded that in this state the pressure gradient must be increased by about 30 times. Consequently, whereas under normal conditions the pressure drop between the aorta and circle of Willis is about 20 mm Hg, during spasm it must be increased to 600 mm Hg, in which case it would be virtually impossible for the blood to flow. The histology of the wall of the internal corotid arteries when fixed in a state of spasm has been studied by Kaufman [245].

In experiments on the internal carotid artery of a dog, isolated *in situ*, the author and his collaborators studied the physiological responses of the wall of this artery to the action of a number of endogenous vasoconstrictor factors in an attempt to elucidate the mechanism of these responses. Comparing the effects of physiologically active vasoconstrictor agents, namely catecholamines, serotonin (serotonin creatine sulfate, Gee Lawson Ltd.), vasopressin (Pitressin, Parke-Davis), and hypertensin (Ciba), showed that serotonin induces constriction of the internal carotid artery in much smaller doses (when its concentration in the perfusion fluid was near to physiological) than catecholamines [257, 300]. When the concentration of serotonin in the perfusion fluid was 0.08 μg/ml, after 10 sec the resistance in the vessel was increased on the average by 3.8 mm Hg/ml/min, and if the sensitivity of the vessel wall was increased, the effect was several times greater. Monoamine oxidase inhibitors, which destroy serotonin, considerably prolonged the constrictor effect of serotonin on the internal carotid artery (Fig. 54). Serotonin could evidently accumulate in the vessel wall and give rise to a prolonged increase in its tone since reserpine (which is known to liberate bound serotonin) led to a prolonged decrease in this tone and to a corresponding decrease in resistance in the internal carotid artery [224, 258] (Fig. 55). Hypertensin, in approximately the same doses as serotonin, can produce a rather less marked constriction of the internal carotid artery in dogs, but characteristically this was accompanied by a habituation effect and the vasoconstriction weakened considerably during subsequent injections of this substance. Vasopressin also produces constriction of the internal carotid artery, but relatively larger doses (0.1-0.01 i.u.) are necessary and, characteristically, the vasoconstrictor effect was much more prolonged and the vasoconstriction resulting from serotonin injected after it also was longer in duration.

Further experiments by the present author and his collaborators showed that an increase in the concentration of potassium ions (at the expense of sodium) during perfusion of the internal carotid artery isolated *in situ* caused rapid contraction of the vessel wall, presumably because of depolarization of the membranes in the smooth-muscle cells of the media. The same effect was given by ouabain,

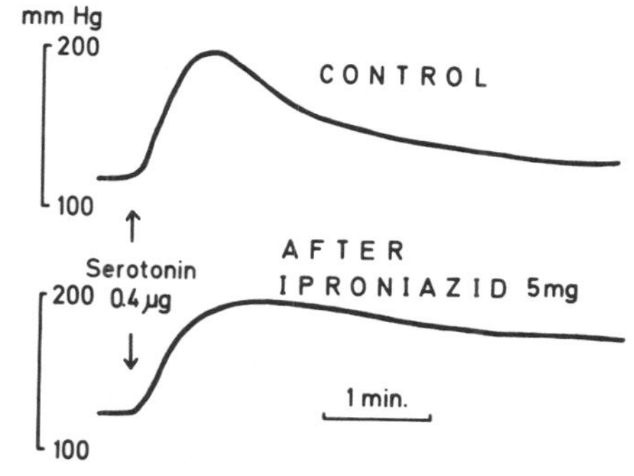

Fig. 54. Change in effect of serotonin on dog's internal carotid artery, isolated *in situ*, after intra-arterial injection of the monoamine oxidase inhibitor iproniazid (5 mg) [224, 258].

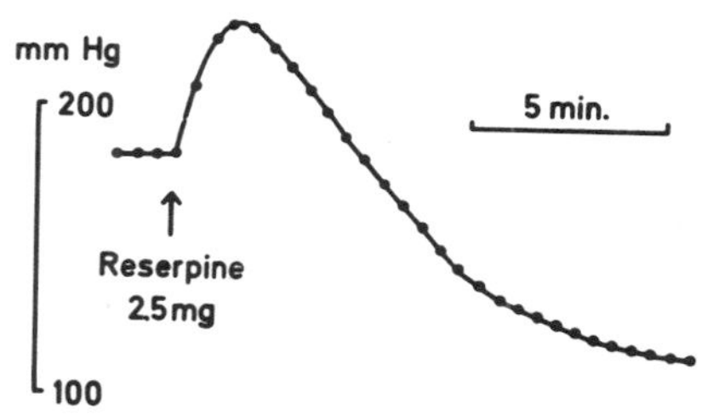

Fig. 55. Effect of reserpine on dog's internal carotid artery, isolated *in situ:* after a temporary increase in resistance in the vessel (evidently because of liberation of bound serotonin and/or catecholamines), marked relaxation of the vessel wall takes place [224, 258].

an inhibitor of sodium-potassium ATPase in the vessel wall, which disturbs active transport of ions, and causes depolarization of the cell membranes. Under these conditions the effect of vasoconstrictor substances, including serotonin, could be greatly increased and prolonged. Calcium ions evidently play an important role in the genesis of the vasoconstrictor effect of serotonin and other constrictor agents on the vessel wall and in maintaining its normal tone [246]. After the corresponding changes leading to the development of spasm had taken place in the vessel wall, constrictor stimuli (for example, the direct action of serotonin) caused it to contract, after which relaxation did not occur, and the staircase phenomena developed (Fig. 56). The resulting spasm was not due to any pathological flow of impulses along vasoconstrictor nerve fibers, for it was not abolished by α-blocking drugs such as dihydroergotoxin. It arose because of changes in the membranes or contractile system of the vessel wall itself, for it was usually abolished by typical myogenic spasmolytics, notably by papaverine (Fig. 57).

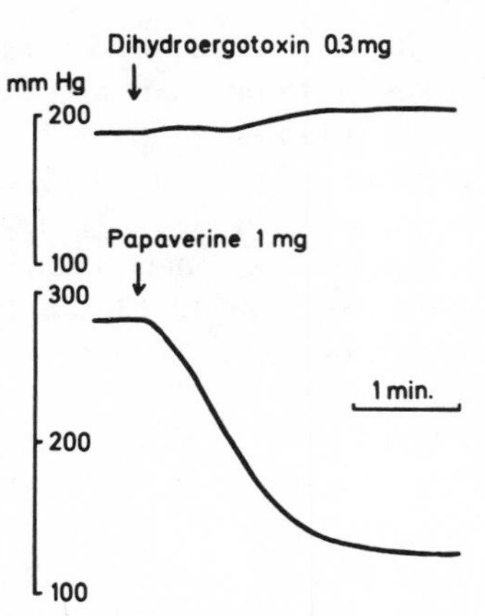

Fig. 57. The α-adrenergic blocking agent dihydroergotoxin does not produce relaxation of the wall of the internal carotid artery, isolated *in situ*, when in a state of spasm, whereas papaverine abolishes the spasm of this vessel [224].

It is thus definitely established that the wall of the internal carotid arteries may be very active and can contract to give a sharp decrease in the lumen of the artery, leading to an enormous increase in its hemodynamic resistance. The main problem in the genesis of spasm of the internal carotid artery is how to explain why the contracted wall does not subsequently relax. According to existing experimental data this may depend a) on the accumulation of serotonin, catecholamines, and possibly other endogenous vasoconstrictor substances in the vessel walls, b) on a disturbance of repolarization of the muscle cell membranes, when because of disturbance of active ion transport, after contraction of the smooth muscle cells K^+ ions do not re-enter the cell, and c) on changes in the contractile mechanism of the myofibrils, so that after contraction they do not relax, although at present the reasons for this disturbance are unknown and call for further investigation.

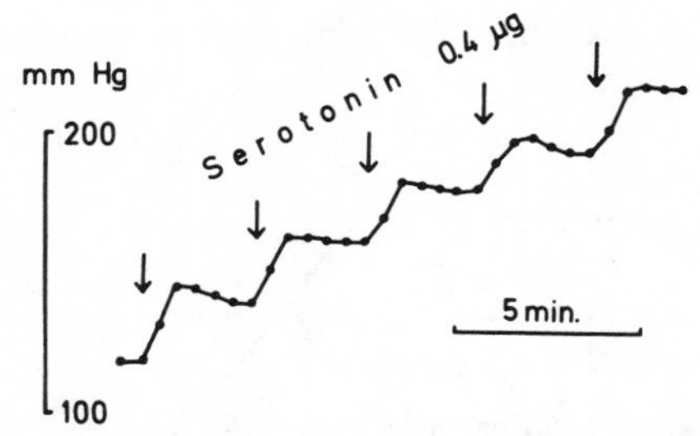

Fig. 56. The "staircase phenomenon" during repeated injections of serotonin into the dog's internal carotid artery isolated *in situ*, when the resistance in the vessel increased stepwise. This phenomenon occurs whenever the alternation of contraction and relaxation in smooth-muscle cells of the vessel wall is disturbed so that they do not relax after contraction, and and vascular spasm develops [224].

When spasm of the internal carotid artery has already developed it is difficult to abolish it because most methods applied have only a temporary effect [241]. In many cases, however, spasm of these arteries can be abolished by local application of substances causing vasodilatation (papaverine etc.). In these experiments the effect varied depending on whether the spasmolytics were injected into the systemic blood stream intravenously or directly into the artery in spasm. Papaverine, for example, when injected intravenously, weakened constriction of the internal carotid arteries to some extent, while at the same time it lowered the systemic arterial pressure. On the one hand, this last effect prevented blood from entering the brain through collateral arteries and, on the other hand, it did not help the flow of blood through the constricted internal carotid artery. When papaverine was injected into the artery, these side-effects did not take place and the spasmolytic effect on the internal carotid arteries was many times stronger. Abolition of spasm of the internal carotid arteries was facilitated by mechanical stretching of the vessel from within by injecting the spasmolytic drugs into it under pressure.

Significant Increase of Resistance in the Very Small Cerebral Vessels as a Cause of Cerebrovascular Disturbances

It was stated above (Chapters II, III, and IV) that a characteristic feature distinguishing the small cortical arteries is the narrowing of their lumen under a variety of conditions. If the decrease in lumen is not very great, because of the short extent of these arteries and the relatively slow blood flow (compared with the pial vessels), as well as because of the Fahraeus–Lindqvist rheologic phenomenon, this does not necessarily increase the vascular resistance. In some cases, however, constriction of the intracerebral vessels, especially of the precapillary arterioles, is so considerable that it cannot but create an obstacle to the movement of erythrocytes, thereby reducing the blood supply to the brain tissue. This can occur in a focus of paroxysmal activity. It has been shown [125, 244] that, after local application of strychnine to the cat cortex, the blood flow in that region is increased on the average by 45%, after which it begins to diminish, although paroxysmal discharges as a rule persisted for much longer (Fig. 58). Comparison showed that the intensity of the circulation was reduced on the average 4 times quicker than the number of paroxysmal cortical discharges (Fig. 59). Usually paroxysmal activity could be detected in the cortex for many minutes after the increase in

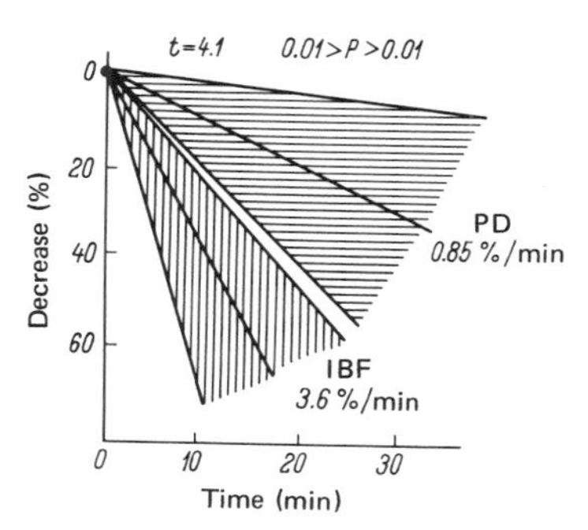

Fig. 59. Mean rate of decrease of paroxysmal discharges (PD, horizontally shaded sector) and of decrease in intensity of blood flow (IBF, vertically shaded sector) in parietal cortex of a cat. Arithmetic mean values and standard deviations are shown [125]. Explanation in text.

blood flow had not only disappeared, but had been followed by a marked decrease below its initial level; in these experiments the blood flow fell on the average to 75 ± 2% of its initial level. Direct experiments thus showed that there is not only a relative, but an absolute deficiency of blood supply in a focus of paroxysmal activity. These findings are in agreement with the results of other investigations [269], in which, despite dilatation of the pial arteries, definite evidence of a deficient blood supply was found in a focus of paroxysmal activity: cyanosis of the vessels on the brain surface, flattening of the electrocorticogram, a decrease in the oxygen tension in the cortex; the illustrations in the paper cited show that the blood flow in the cortex, measured by means of thermistors, was increased only when the systemic arterial pressure was raised. These observations are confirmed by other studies [292] showing that the vascular density can decrease appreciably in cortical regions exhibiting paroxysmal discharges.

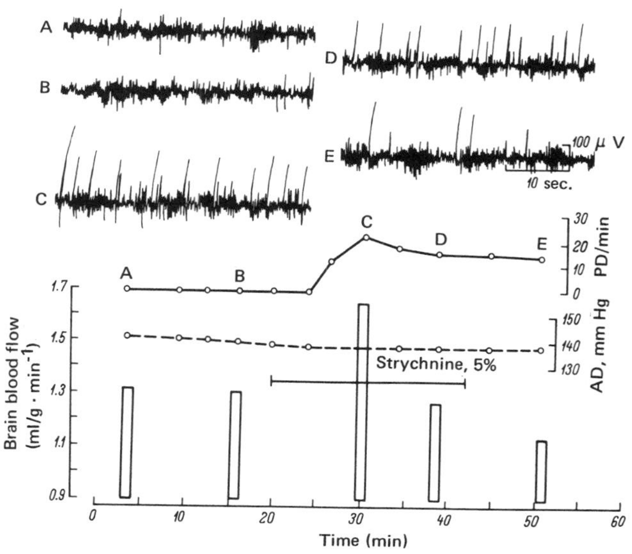

Fig. 58. Changes in regional blood flow and paroxysmal activity produced by strychnine application to the cerebral cortex of a cat. Upper half of figure: patterns of EEG at moments A, B, C, D, and E [125, 244].

The writer's subsequent investigations showed that the most probable cause of this deficiency of cortical blood supply in a focus of paroxysmal activity is a sudden constriction of the lumen of the smallest intracerebral vessels, for under those conditions the systemic arterial pressure and the state of the major arteries of the brain remained unchanged [212], and the pial arteries were actually dilated [218, 250]. Vital fixation of the vessel walls in the cerebral cortex at various times after local application of strychnine, followed by measurement of the lumen of a large number of cortical vessels

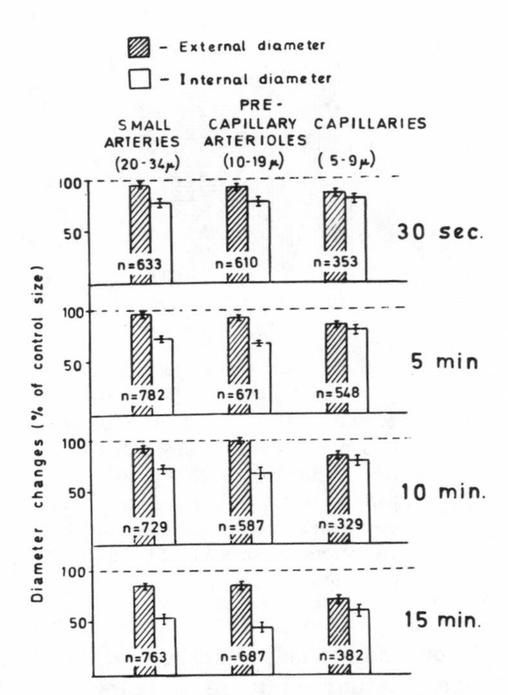

Fig. 60. Changes in diameter of cortical blood vessels in rabbits after strychnine applications of different duration to the cortex. Results (mean values and mean errors) are given in percentage of vascular diameters in control experiments [244].

in microscopic sections not only revealed the direction of the vascular responses, but also made it possible to study the dynamics of changes in these responses at different times after application of strychnine [235, 244]. Within a few minutes after application of strychnine, constriction of the cortical vessels began, and then continued to increase in severity (Fig. 60). This narrowing of the lumen of the cortical vessels in a focus of paroxysmal activity was accompanied by definite microscopic changes in the vessel walls. Changes in the muscle cells, which appeared morphologically to be constricted [244] and bulged into the lumen of the vessel (Fig. 61, A, B), could be seen as early as 30 sec after application of strychnine. After a longer action of strychnine (5-10 min), the media of the cortical arteries in places began to separate longitudinally into layers (Fig. 61 C, D), and subsequently these changes increased in degree, so that the wall appeared to be homogenized and thickened, narrowing the lumen irregularly. During a paroxysmal state, changes in the muscle cells of the cortical arteries and arterioles, leading to narrowing their lumen, were thus the most conspicuous feature.

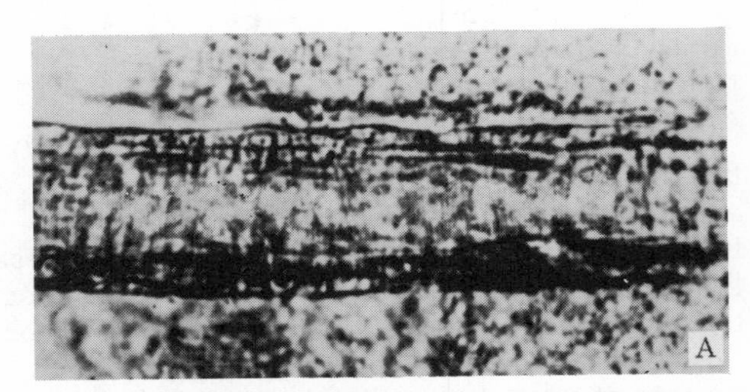

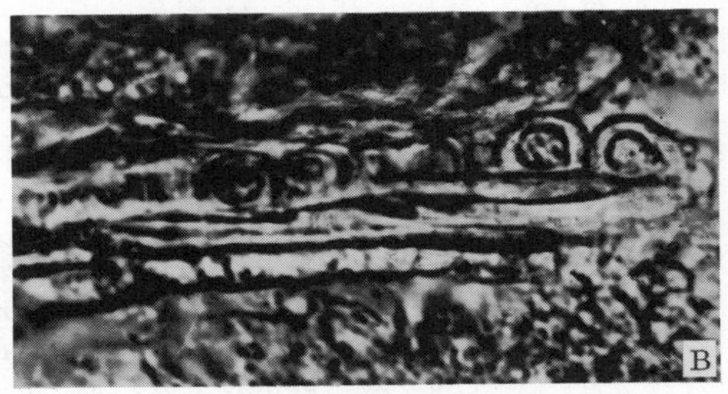

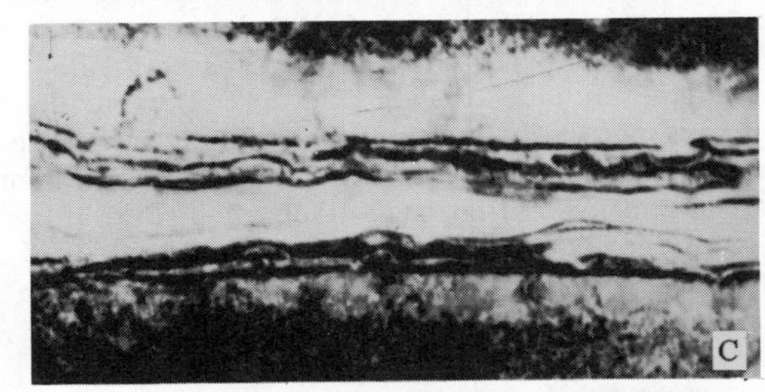

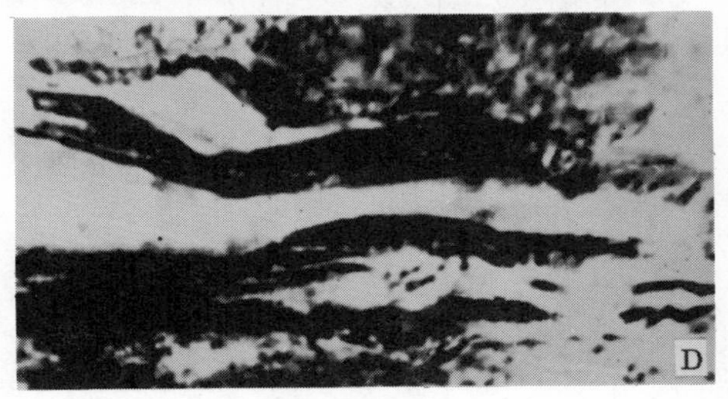

Fig. 61. Histological changes in walls of cortical arteries in the brain of rabbits during paroxysmal activity [235]. Photomicrographs of unstained sections, unretouched: A) cortical artery during absence of paroxysmal activity (control) 630X; B) swelling of muscle cells and thickening of vessel walls, leading to constriction of lumen, 900X; C) longitudinal separation of media of small artery into layers, 630X; D) intramural spaces formed through separation of media of a cortical artery into layers, 630X.

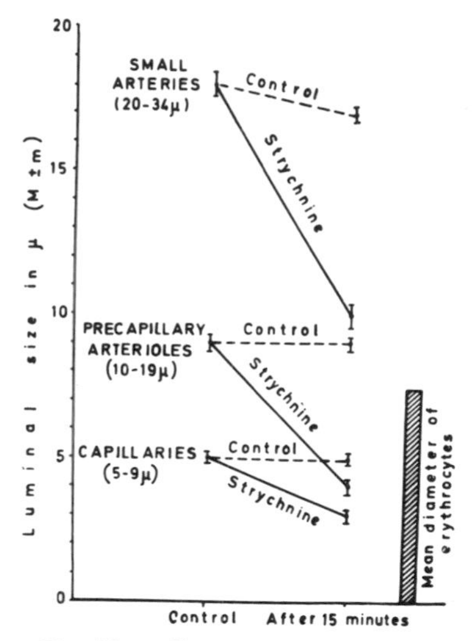

Fig. 62. Differences in narrowing of lumen of cortical blood vessels in experiments with strychnine application for 15 min compared with control (experiments of same duration; no strychnine applied; exposure of cortex only). Both mean values and mean errors are given. Diagram is based upon 4839 measurements of diameter [244].

As was mentioned above, during a gradual narrowing of the lumen of these small vessels, the fluidity of blood in them increases until the erythrocytes start to jam inside the vessel [129]. The results of measurement of the diameter of the cortical arteries, given in Fig. 62, show that the cortical precapillary arteries from 20 to 34 μ in diameter are not constricted sufficiently for erythrocytes to jam in them, despite the marked contraction of their lumen down to half its initial level. In the case of the precapillary arterioles (10-19 μ) and capillaries (5-9 μ), on the other hand, the result of contraction of their lumen by 50% or more was that even deformed (i.e., elongated) erythrocytes should be unable to pass through them. This cannot but create a considerable resistance to the blood flow in the focus of paroxysmal activity and to lead ultimately to deficiency of its blood supply, despite the continued high level of electrical activity and the occurrence of paroxysmal discharges in the electrocorticogram.

An increase of resistance in the smallest blood vessels of the brain causing slowing of the blood flow can also be produced by *increased intravascular aggregation of erythrocytes*. This phenomenon has been studied in detail during the last 25 years, but in other organs of animals and man and not in the brain. On the one hand, increased aggregation of erythrocytes arising during various diseases and under various conditions has been studied [152, 27, 104, 151], and the results have shown that such aggregates can obstruct arterioles and thus prevent blood from flowing into the capillary network. Increased aggregation of erythrocytes taking place within capillaries of a small vascular bed, and giving rise to such a high resistance to the blood flow in the capillaries that it is retarded, or even stopped completely (stasis), has also been investigated [204, 208].

Intravascular aggregation of erythrocytes, which was observed simultaneously with slowing of the blood flow and interruption of the column of erythrocytes in the vessels, has been described in direct biomicroscopic investigations of the circulation on the brain surface in small pial arteries [270]. Slowing of the blood flow reached such a degree that complete stasis developed. In these experiments the erythrocyte sedimentation rate in vitro was increased. These phenomena were seen particularly clearly after the eating of fat, or especially, after intravenous injection of macromolecular polysaccharides and various plasma substitutes [400]. The same workers observed that if foci of ischemia were present, following occlusion of the afferent arteries, the appearance of intravascular aggregation of erythrocytes led to still further slowing of the blood flow [401].

In cerebral edema, stasis has been observed in the capillaries in pathomorphological investigations [360]. To determine whether the appearance of stasis in edema is connected with increased intravascular aggregation of the erythrocytes, their aggregation was investigated in the present author's experiments on dogs in blood taken from the sagittal sinus of the brain (i.e., in blood which had just flowed through the brain capillaries [227, 229]). The intensity of aggregation of the erythrocytes was determined from the erythrocyte sedimentation rate, using blood from the femoral vein as the control.* These experiments showed that, if cerebral edema developed rapidly (within approximately 10 min) the erythrocyte sedimentation rate in blood taken from the vein was unchanged, even though the degree of prolapse was very considerable. If, however, the edema developed comparatively slowly, the sedimentation rate of erythrocytes in blood which had just flowed through the brain capillaries was con-

*A similar method was used by investigators studying other organs [412].

siderably increased. This indicated that intravascular aggregation of the erythrocytes in the brain also was increased. This aggregation was so marked that clumps of erythrocytes could be seen with the unaided eye in upright pipets. Increased intravascular aggregation of erythrocytes as discovered in the brain during cerebral edema, may also be found in other types of cerebrovascular pathology, although this problem is still virtually unstudied.

Double Significance of Some Compensatory Responses in Cerebrovascular Disorders

The function of compensatory mechanisms in certain cerebrovascular disorders was examined in Chapters II and III. Despite the sophisticated regulation and high powers of compensation possessed by the cerebral circulation, its disorders frequently cannot be overcome and prove fatal to life. This may partly be explained by the fact that in many cases there are two types of disturbances in the brain: on the one hand a deficiency of the blood supply and on the other hand, cerebral edema. Operation of the compensatory mechanisms reducing the deficiency of blood supply increases the cerebral edema, and conversely, if they reduce the edema, they increase the circulatory deficiency. This not only prevents the natural protective adaptations of the body from overcoming the cerebrovascular disorder, but it also places difficulties in the way of the development of prophylactic and therapeutic clinical measures.

For instance, it was stated above that following occlusion of the cranial vena cava, the cerebrovascular disorders and their sequelae (deficient blood supply and cerebral edema) are compensated in the brain by the system of the internal carotid and vertebral arteries, the pial arteries, the veins, and also through changes in the systemic arterial pressure [232]. However, the vascular reactions described above cannot diminish the severity of cerebrovascular disorders to any considerable degree: if they remove some disorders they help to produce others (Table 5). A reflex diminution of the systemic arterial pressure after occlusion of the cranial vena cava (restricting the development of edema), for instance, must slow the blood flow in the cerebrovascular system and increase the deficiency of the blood supply. The same remarks apply to constriction of the major arteries of the brain, reducing the pressure gradient in the cerebral vessels. On the other hand, the elevation

TABLE 5. Role of Compensatory Responses in the Development of Edema and of a Deficiency of Blood Supply of the Brain after Occlusion of the Cranial Vena Cava (+ Denotes a Positive, – a Negative Role from the Point of View of Removing the Pathological Changes)

Compensatory responses	Effect on cerebral edema	Effect on deficiency of blood supply to brain
Collateral drainage of blood into system of caudal vena cava	+	+
Reduction of systemic arterial pressure during occlusion	+	–
Elevation of systemic arterial pressure after reopening of vena cava	–	+
Constriction of major arteries of the brain (internal carotid and vertebral arteries)	+	–
Dilatation of pial arteries	–	+

of the systemic arterial pressure after removal of the occlusion, and also the dilatation of the pial arteries, aimed at overcoming the deficiency of the blood supply must increase the blood pressure in the capillaries of the brain, accelerate the formation of edema, and delay its absorption.

The double role of these compensatory phenomena in the brain can also be seen in the case of occlusion of the aorta [231]. Besides the deficiency of blood supply to the brain, a constant complication of this condition is cerebral edema, which actually begins to develop during the occlusion but increases sharply in severity after its removal. Possible causes of the cerebral edema in this case are, first, the changes in the capillary walls and surrounding brain tissue due to ischemia and, second, elevation of the venous and, consequently, the intracapillary pressure in the brain. Immediately after removal of the occlusion from the aorta and restoration of its patency, the cerebral edema increases sharply. The reason for this is clear: not only does the arterial pressure rise to its initial level when this is done, but becomes higher still, and biomicroscopic investigations of vessels on the surface of the brain have shown that the blood flow in them is quickly restored and the blood pressure in the cerebral capillaries must rise. The compensatory reactions which remove the manifestations of cerebral ischemia (elevation of the blood pressure in the capillaries and increased permeability of their walls) thus give rise to a second pathological state: to cerebral edema and swelling. Constriction of the major arteries of the brain at this period, although undoubtedly beneficial from the point of view of limiting the development of edema, at the same time delays the correction of cerebral ischemia, because it reduces the pressure gradient in the vessels of the brain and causes a relative decrease in the inflow of blood into its capillaries.

This dual nature of the compensatory responses, i.e., their positive yet, at the same time, negative role, places the clinician in a dilemma: how can the normal brain function be preserved; what is to be done so that the maximal benefit and the minimal harm is obtained from each compensatory reaction? The methods used in clinical practice will be most effective if, on the one hand, the fullest possible information is available on what is happening with the patient's cerebral circulation and, on the other hand, if the mechanism of action of the methods used is fully understood, for the possibility cannot be ruled out that, besides their beneficial effect, they may also have a harmful effect.

CHAPTER V

ORGANIZATION OF THE VASCULAR MECHANISMS

The investigations listed in the previous chapters have shed light on the functional organization of the vascular system of the brain [220, 222]. By functional organization of the vascular system of the brain in this case is meant the general principles governing the functional behavior of its different parts under conditions when the cerebral circulation is regulated. The different parts of the cerebral arterial system naturally deserve special interest, because it is this system that is the chief hemodynamic operator regulating the inflow of blood into the capillary network and the changes in the capillary circulation.

The problem of the functional organization of the vascular system of the brain could be analyzed only by systematic research into every aspect of the functional behavior of different parts of the cerebrovascular system. Such investigations have revealed the significance of various parts of the cerebrovascular system, on the one hand, in producing changes in the capillary circulation, i.e., in the intensity of the blood supply to the brain tissues in the strict meaning of the term, and on the other hand, in compensating cerebrovascular disturbances.

As a result of these investigations different patterns of functional behavior (as regards regulation of the cerebral circulation) were discovered in at least four different parts of the arterial system of the brain (the major trunks, the pial, precortical, and intracerebral arteries) and in two parts of the venous system (the pial veins and the emissary veins of the skull). These parts of the vascular system of the brain may behave differently, as regards the characteristic direction of their responses (constriction or dilatation), depending on the kind of regulation of the cerebral circulation. Under different concrete conditions the responses may be either concerted or relatively independent.

Though the majority of the experimental findings concerning the functional behavior of the major arteries of the brain have been obtained in experiments on rabbits and dogs, it can be assumed that this vascular mechanism is very active in all animals from those at the lower levels of development of the vascular system of the brain to man. In amphibians (frogs), for instance, in which the function of the major arteries of the brain is performed by the internal cerebral arteries, Ormotsadze has shown that a segment of this artery can constrict under various conditions and can thereby regulate the inflow of blood to the brain [223, 299]. On the other hand, in the more highly developed vertebrates such as monkeys, active responses of the internal carotid arteries have also been found [332]. As was mentioned above (Chapter IV), active constriction of the internal carotid arteries resembling spasm has also been seen in man. Consequently, the role of the major arteries of the brain in regulating the cerebral circulation, as well as in the genesis of its disturbances, has been demonstrated in the majority of the vertebrates, including man. This function is apparently present also in animals in which the internal carotid arteries have become obliterated and the carotid system supplies blood to the circle of Willis via branches of the external carotid artery and the rete mirabile located inside the bone; this, as we know, is the case in cats.

The next problem is to identify the segments of the major arteries of the brain where constriction may occur, i.e., where the "closing mechanism" is located. To examine this problem, initially a fixing solution (20% formalin in alcohol) was injected intra-arterially under standard conditions into living rabbits and dogs. The subsequent study of serial sections, and also of casts of the vessels, revealed constriction of the internal carotid arteries, mainly in the winding part of their course within the cavernous sinuses [209], and of the vertebral arteries.

Similar results were recently obtained in experiments on dogs in which the author and his coworkers successfully fixed the walls of the internal carotid arteries during spasm caused by depolarization of their muscular layer [245]. Characteristically, constriction of the major arteries of the brain was frequently not concentric: in places the walls projected into the lumen of the vessel, which became stellate or flattened in shape. This must presumably be of considerable physiological importance, because flattening of the lumen of a vessel causes a sharp increase in the intravascular resistance [345].

These considerable changes in shape of the vascular lumen (local invaginations, twistings, and so on) were bound to give rise to turbulences in the flow of blood, although the resistance to the blood flow could not have been greatly increased. The muscular layer of this artery inside the bone is about about twice as thick as in the intracranial portions (although the workers who described this phenomenon [145] directed attention only to the presence of elastic fibers in the vessel wall within the bone). Recent histological investigations of the walls of the internal carotid arteries in dogs [245] have shown that these vessels are of the muscular type with 10-20 layers of smooth-muscle fibers which, under ordinary conditions, are arranged predominantly circularly. During contraction of the wall, the inner elastic membrane becomes highly folded, and in places it becomes double, while pulvinate swellings project from the vessel wall into its lumen.

Along the course of the internal and carotid and vertebral arteries in some vertebrates and in man there are distinct curvatures situated, in the case of the carotid arteries, usually within the cavernous sinus. The following physiological functions have been ascribed to these curvatures: a) damping the pulse waves of the blood pressure [148], which are much greater in the aorta than in the circle of Willis; b) facilitating the outflow of venous blood from the skull, because the curvatures of the major arteries pulsate inside the venous sinuses, where valves, which are assumed to prevent the reflux of blood into the skull [369, 29], have been described at the sites where the veins enter them; c) the production of eddies in the blood flow [372] and d) the evidently substantial changes in resistance even in the presence of only slight changes in the lumen of the blood vessels.

The major arteries of the brain undoubtedly constitute a functionally united system. Indeed, it cannot be otherwise, because of the existence of these extensive anastomoses between them in the region of the circle of Willis, although the functional behavior of these arteries does show certain peculiarities. Thus it was observed [242, 243] that the width of their lumen can fluctuate periodically, and these fluctuations are reciprocal in character: while one artery dilates, another constricts, and vice versa (Fig. 69, Chapter VI). Because of this, the resultant effect of the functional behavior of the major arteries of the brain, as reflected in the intensity of the blood inflow into the circle of Willis and in the level of the blood pressure therein, may remain unchanged and can thus ensure a constant blood supply to the brain. Investigations by other workers [169], who measured the blood flow simultaneously in the internal carotid and vertebral arteries by means of Rein's thermostromuhr, showed that in certain types of shock the changes in blood flow in these arteries do not run parallel. However, not all the lateral branches and anastomoses of these arteries with the extracranial vessels were ligated, and this could obviously have exerted a profound effect on the results of measurement.

It has now been proved that the system of major arteries of the brain regulates a constant inflow of blood into the circle of Willis. On the one hand, the pulse, respiratory, and other relatively rapid fluctuations of the systemic arterial pressure are damped in these arteries. On the other hand, because of the manner in which the arteries function, a constant inflow of blood into the circle of Willis is maintained during prolonged changes in the level of the systemic arterial pressure, i.e., the autoregulation of the cerebral circulation is accomplished.

During disturbances of the circulation in the brain as a whole, when there is no primary or clearly defined deficiency of blood supply to the brain tissue, i.e., during a relatively slight and transient stagnation of blood in the venous system of the brain, and also during traumatic edema, active constriction of the major arteries of the brain is observed. Since the circulatory disturbances which develop in the brain may thereby become weakened or abolished, this vasoconstriction can be regarded as a compensatory phenomenon.

The same effect is found during other changes in the cerebral circulation, when there is a tendency for the brain to become congested with blood or for edema to form (severe venous stagnation, postischemic states, general asphyxia), along with a deficiency in the blood supply to the brain. It can accordingly be concluded that the major arteries of the brain have their own laws of functional behavior distinguishing them from the pial arteries, they participate only in the compensation of general disturbances of the cerebral circulation regardless of whether their constriction is of negative value from the point of view of overcoming the deficient blood supply to the brain or not.

Consequently, while it plays an important role in regulating the inflow of blood inside the skull in disturbances arising outside the brain, and also in the compensation of some general disorders of the circulation in the whole brain, the system of major arteries of the brain does not participate, according to existing experimental data, in regulating the adequate inflow of blood into the brain tissue in the case of changes in its metabolic requirements.

Most methods used to study the function of the major arteries of the brain (Chapter I) reveal the functional behavior of the internal carotid and vertebral arteries, but do not give evidence of the responses of the circle of Willis or the other large arteries at the base of the brain. However, this still does not mean that other arteries lying at the base of the brain do not also help to regulate the cerebral circulation. Unfortunately, these vessels are difficult of access for intravital investigation, but evidence of their active role in this regulation is given, first, by the cuff-like thickenings in the walls of these arteries at the base of the brain discovered by morphologists [177, 94]; second, by the high reactivity of their walls, for they contract sharply in response to mechanical stimulation [313]; and third, by the gradual transition between the functional properties of the major arteries of the brain and those of the pial arteries which becomes apparent when the former are constricted while the latter are dilated. For example, during occlusion of the cranial vena cava in dogs the large pial arteries (branches of the middle cerebral artery) react to begin with like the major arteries of the brain, but during repeated occlusions they react like the pial arteries [232]. Consequently, from the functional standpoint, the large pial arteries were found to occupy an intermediate position between the major arteries of the brain and the smaller pial arteries.

Although the muscular layer in the walls of the pial arteries is comparatively thin [294], it can alter the lumen of the vessel actively within wide limits. Considerable constriction of the pial arteries appears in response to direct mechanical or electrical stimulation, but under more natural conditions only comparatively slight constriction of these vessels is observed. This occurs in general circulatory disturbances in the brain when there is no primary deficiency of its blood supply, such as in traumatic cerebral edema and when slight venous stagnation is present in the brain. However, investigations of these vessels under a wide range of different conditions have shown that the typical response of the pial arteries is by dilatation: in every case when the balance between the existing blood supply and the metabolic requirements of the brain tissue is disturbed (during a sharp increase in its activity or when the inflow of blood into it is reduced), as a rule the pial arteries dilate, restoring an adequate circulation. The pial arteries also dilate when the blood supply is deficient, such as during severe venous stasis and also when a deficient blood supply is associated with various types of congestion of the cerebral vessels and with edema (for example, in postischemic states and in general asphyxia), when the system of the major arteries, on the other hand, is constricted as it performs a different function (see above). These facts indicate that the basic rule governing the functional behavior of the pial arteries during regulation of the cerebral circulation is its participation in overcoming the deficiency of blood supply to the brain tissue, regardless of the causes responsible for it; moreover, this rule of functional behavior is seen particularly clearly in the case of the small pial arteries (less than $100\,\mu$ in diameter in rabbits), for their dilatation in the presence of a deficient blood supply to the cortex was always more marked in the small than in the large pial arteries [232, 240, 250, 253].

The functional behavior of arteries located in the substance of the cerebral cortex, between the pial arteries and the cortical capillary network, remained unknown for a long time. This is because intravital observations on these vessels are impossible and also because no other methods of investigating their functions were then available. It was only several years ago that it became possible to investigate the behavior of these arteries during changes in the cerebral circulation. Experiments on rabbits showed that, with an increase in the CO_2 concentration in the inspired air and in the blood circulating in the cerebral vessels, and also if the metabolic needs of the brain tissue were increased (in a postischemic state or during greatly increased brain activity), although when the pial arteries were regularly dilated, thus increasing the circulation in the cortex, the cortical arteries and arterioles remained undilated. Measurements of the external diameter of the cortical arteries under the same conditions revealed only slight variations, not exceeding a few percent compared with the control [234, 238]. At the same time the lumen of these arteries, whatever their caliber, was consistently decreased. At first glance, this constriction of the small cortical arteries, other conditions being equal, should have increased the resistance to the blood flow and thereby reduced the intensity of the capillary circulation in the corresponding zones of the cortex.

However, the actual increase in blood flow in these regions of the brain was evidence that where marked dilatation of the pial arteries took place simultaneously, the total resistance in the cerebral vessels was reduced. This undoubtedly is explained by the special role of the pial arteries in changes in cerebrovascular resistance.

When the responsibility of the pial and cortical arteries for cerebrovascular resistance is examined, two problems must evidently be distinguished: first, the contribution of each group of vessels under stationary conditions to the total absolute resistance, and second, the effect of dilatation and constriction of the pial and cortical arteries on the change in this resistance during regulation of the cortical blood flow.

Investigations on rabbits have shown that the pial arteries, which participate particularly actively in regulation of the cortical blood flow, are between 40 and 100 μ in diameter, while the cortical arteries in these animals are less than 40 μ in diameter. Remembering that according to Poiseuille's formula (if it is considered that this applies to the blood flow in the microcirculatory system), resistance is inversely proportional to the fourth power of the radius of the vessels, it can be concluded that, other conditions being equal, the absolute resistance in the pial arteries is much smaller than in the cortical arteries. However, judging by the other parameters, the resistance in the pial arteries must be (other conditions being equal) higher than in the cortical arteries, since: a) the velocity of the blood flow (which is inversely proportional to the resistance) must be greater in the pial arteries than in the cortical, for in the transition from the first to the second the total area of cross section of the lumina of the vessels is increased; b) the length of the vessels (to which their resistance is directly proportional) is as follows: the total duration of the pial arteries, according to the author's measurements, is 40 times greater in rabbits than in that of the cortical arteries and arterioles (in larger animals this difference must be correspondingly greater); and c) according to the Fahraeus–Lindqvist phenomenon, the narrower the lumen of the vessels, the smaller the relative viscosity of the blood in them, if their caliber is below 100 μ [66, 406, 129, 108, 35, 36], i.e., it must be greater in the pial than in the cortical arteries. Direct evidence that the pial arteries in fact play an important role in creating the absolute magnitude of the cerebrovascular resistance is given by recently published [53] direct measurements of the pressure in the pial arteries, showing that along the length of these vessels (until they enter the cortex) it falls to 50% of the systemic arterial pressure, while according to measurements made by other workers [374], it falls to 60%.

So far as the changes in hemodynamic resistance in the pial and cortical arteries during functional hyperemia in the cortex are concerned, such as, for example, when its activity is stimulated by strychnine, the small pial arteries were dilated on the average by 45%, while the cortical arteries constricted (initially) by only 15%, i.e., by an amount three times smaller. Further, considering that the great length of the pial arteries, it can be concluded that any considerable dilatation of them must reduce this resistance very substantially. Finally, the rheologic features of the blood flow in the microvascular system must play an important role in the changes in resistance under the conditions specified above: because of the Fahraeus–Lindqvist effect, with a decrease in the lumen of such small blood vessels, the flowability of the blood in them cannot be reduced, but may even be increased [225]. Consequently, this explains why the slight constriction of the comparatively short cortical arteries does not prevent an increase in the circulation in the cortex under all the conditions specified above.

The functional behavior of the pial and cortical arteries corresponds to their anatomy. The pial arteries lie on the surface of the cerebral hemispheres in the relatively wide canals of the subarachnoid space and are supported inside them by bands of connective tissue connecting the vascular walls with the walls of the canals [14]. The pial arteries are thus surrounded entirely by cerebrospinal fluid; this is under comparatively low pressure and can travel freely in the subarachnoid spaces. Under these conditions the pial arteries can dilate to any degree, thus increasing the inflow of blood into the cortex should the increased metabolic needs so require. So far as the smaller arteries lying within the cortex are concerned, according to the experimental findings mentioned above they do not dilate even when the cortical circulation is significantly increased. This is evidently of special functional importance. The walls of the cortical arteries are covered externally by connective-tissue and glial structures, which connect them to the surrounding tissue elements of the brain. Electron-microscopic investigations [189, 305] have shown that there is almost no free space around the walls of the intracerebral arteries, so that any dilatation of these vessels must exert a mechanical effect upon the surrounding neurons, displacing and compressing them. In fact, however, this does not happen: the external diameter of the cortical arteries does not increase under different circumstances, and as to the regular decrease in the lumen of the cortical arteries under all the conditions listed it is apparently the characteristic functional behavior of these blood vessels, although the physiological significance and mechanism of its origin are still obscure.

Vascular responses of different parts of the arterial system of the brain under various conditions are shown in Table 6.

The microcirculation of blood in the capillaries within the brain substance still awaits investigation, for although most of the methods used until recently to investigate the capillary system of the brain reflected its morphology, they did not shed light on the behavior of the capillary circulation during various types of circulatory changes in different parts of the brain.

Injection of the vascular system with contrast materials simply enables the anatomy of the intracerebral vessels to be studied [308, 295, 60]. Histological investigations with selective staining of the erythrocytes (for example, with benzidine or acid fuchsin), when the brain was fixed after the animal's death, were unsuitable for this purpose because they may be accompanied by displacement of blood, aggregation of erythrocytes inside the vessels, and so on; the pictures thus obtained can therefore differ sharply from those actually found during life. Impregnation of the walls of the cerebral vessels with silver [147, 148] enables open, "closed," and growing capillaries to be stained. However, this method does not enable open capillaries to be differentiated into those which are active (filled with whole blood) and those filled with plasma and representing an intermediate stage between active and closed capillaries [208, 226]; furthermore, prolonged preliminary treatment of the tissue and the silver precipitated during impregnation on the walls of the capillaries are bound to distort the true di-

TABLE 6. Responses of Various Vascular Mechanisms of the Brain under Different Conditions

	Primary changes in systemic arterial pressure		Disturbances in whole brain; congestion of vessels, venous stagnation, cerebral edema		Disturbances of blood supply in small areas of the brain	
			without primary deficiency of blood supply	with deficiency of blood supply to brain tissue	Primary disturbances of blood supply	Increased activity
Conditions studied	Arterial hypertension	Arterial hypotension	1) Traumatic edema 2) Occlusion of cervical veins	1) Occlusion of cranial vena cava 2) Asphyxia 3) Postischemic states	Occlusion of pial arteries	Local application of strychnine
Major brain arteries	Constriction	Dilatation	Constriction	Constriction	No response	No response
Pial arteries	Constriction	Dilatation	Weak Constriction	Dilatation	Dilatation	Dilatation
Precortical arteries	Constriction	No response	? (not studied)	? (not studied)	? (not studied)	? (not studied)
Cortical arteries	? (not studied)	No response	? (not studied)	Narrowing of lumen	? (not studied)	Narrowing of lumen

ameter of the capillaries. When writers who have used these methods have described changes in the width of capillaries [261, 411], it is impossible to be sure that the results obtained reflected the true state of affairs quantitatively.

In view of the impossibility of making intravital observations on the capillary circulation in the brain substance, the writer decided to use a method which reveals some features of the circulation in microscopic specimens [206]. After the development of particular changes in the cerebral circulation, the cortex of a rabbit was fixed intravitally through the pia and arachnoid (after removal of bone and of the dura), with a 20% solution of formalin (see Chapter I). The number of active capillaries at the time of fixation of the brain per unit of brain volume is

Traumatic cerebral edema	5.8 ± 0.4
Ligation of both carotid arteries	8.2 ± 0.3
Control	9.1 ± 0.3
Inhalation of gas mixture with 10% CO_2	10.3 ± 0.4
Asphyxia (2 min)	13.7 ± 0.4
Aseptic leptomeningitis	14.0 ± 0.4
Injection of cerebral vessels with ink – gelatin mass	10.1 ± 0.5
Impregnation of capillaries with silver by Klosovskii's method	19.1 ± 0.4

The numbers of capillaries detected by injection or silver impregnation, as given above, are much greater than those discovered during changes in the cerebral circulation. At the same time among the many hundreds of capillaries in sections impregnated with silver only a very few "closed" capillaries were found (this is also supported by the observations of Klosovskii himself and of his collaborators). It could thus be assumed that by far the majority of nonfunctioning capillaries in the cerebral cortex (if not all) are filled with plasma [208]. If so, this would be of great physiological significance: in an organ like the brain, it may become necessary to convert nonfunctioning capillaries suddenly into active; opening of the closed capillaries could undoubtedly retard this process [97]. It is interesting to note that in the retina, where the circulation in many respects is evidently similar to the cerebral circulation, only some capillaries (about 30%) have been found filled with whole blood, i.e., are active, while the rest contain only blood plasma [381].

The active role of the veins in regulation of the cerebral circulation is very difficult to detect. Usually their diameter changes more or less passively with changes in the intravascular pressure and in the hemodynamics of the venous circulation. However, it was shown that in traumatic cerebral edema, for instance, the pial veins (in dogs and rabbits) are constricted on the average by 13% [229]. This was not due to mechanical compression of the veins because of the increased intracranial pressure, since it was observed also after extensive trephining of the skull, when the intracranial pressure was equal to zero, although constriction of the veins could be the result of changes in intravascular pressure because of constriction of the major and pial arteries. The active role of the pial veins has so far been demonstrated only after occlusion of the cranial (superior) vena cava in dogs. Serial photomicrography showed that after occlusion, pial veins with a diameter of 120-225 μ were dilated on the average by 15% of their initial diameter; subsequently they began to constrict although the blood pressure in the pial veins remained high (Fig. 19). This was observed even when the skull was widely trephined and the pressure on the pial vessels from outside was not raised. Consequently, the phenomenon described was considered to be an active response of the intracranial veins, evidently leading to a partial decrease in volume of the brain when swollen as a result of edema [232].

Evidence was also obtained of active constriction of the system of emissary veins of the skull conveying blood from the sinuses of the brain into the extracranial venous system. As a result of this constriction of these veins in terminal states [213] and after occlusion of the aorta [231], the blood pressure in the veins and also, evidently, in the capillaries of the brain rose, and thus could partly overcome the severe deficiency of the blood supply to the brain under these conditions, enabling substances to be transported from the blood vessels to the extracellular spaces and to the tissue elements of the brain.

The venous system of the brain thus can also participate actively in the regulation of the cerebral circulation, by compensating some of its disturbances. However, this takes place only under severe pathological conditions, when the functional behavior of the vascular mechanisms of the cerebral arterial system cannot overcome the severe disturbances of the circulation in the brain.

The investigations so far carried out have thus elucidated the general principles governing the functional behavior of the different vascular mechanisms of the brain. They also explain the functional organization of the arterial system of the brain regulating the cerebral circulation under normal and pathological conditions.

PART 2

PHYSIOLOGICAL MECHANISMS OF FUNCTIONAL BEHAVIOR OF THE CEREBRAL ARTERIES

CHAPTER VI

THE MAJOR ARTERIES

As a whole the physiological mechanisms of functional behavior of the main arteries (like other arteries) of the brain are much less understood than the functional behavior of the vascular mechanisms of the brain under different conditions described in the first part of this book. The reason is not so much that fewer investigations have been made of these problems, but that most work so far published has been carried out without any attempt to analyze functional differences between different parts of the cerebrovascular system. Only the blood flow or the total cerebrovascular resistance was recorded in them, and consequently, the problems could not be attacked from the aspect with which we are concerned in this book.

The signals determining the physiological behavior of the major arteries (internal carotid and vertebral) when regulating the cerebral circulation under normal and pathological conditions may arise as feedbacks by a variety of humoral and neural mechanisms. In addition, purely mechanical (hemodynamic) mechanisms may also operate. These may be changes in the resistance in blood vessels making comparatively complex twists and turns along their course, changes in the velocity of the blood flow in them, and direct myogenic responses of the smooth-muscle layer of the arterial wall to changes in intravascular pressure.

Direct Effects of Physiologically Active Substances on the Internal Carotid Arteries

Among the various humoral factors circulating in the blood and manifesting their effects directly on the walls of the major arteries of the brain, hormones or neurohumors are of particular interest. Investigations in the last decade have demonstrated the high sensitivity of the major arteries of the brain to the action of physiologically active substances. In the original investigations of the author and his associates the vascular system of the brain was undisturbed, and when small doses of these substances were injected into one of the major arteries of the brain, with all the other arteries remaining intact, responses of the internal carotid arteries were judged from changes in the blood flow in them [242, 90, 241]. Later investigations demonstrated the great advantages of working with the isolated internal carotid arteries of dogs *in situ* (see Chapter I). Responses of the vessel wall were found to persist even after exclusion of the anastomoses which connect these vessels to branches of the internal maxillary arteries. The sensitivity of the walls of the internal carotid arteries to physiologically active substances (such as noradrenalin, acetylcholine, serotonin, vasopressin, etc.) was found to be significantly high. When the perfusion pressure was recorded in the isolated internal carotid artery *in situ*, the resistance in that vessel was found to vary within wide limits. It could be increased so much that the blood would stop in the vessel despite a very high perfusion pressure (300 mm Hg or more).

During light anesthesia the isolated internal carotid arteries actually respond to small doses (0.1-0.5 μg) of physiologically active substances when injected intra-arterially: noradrenalin and acetylcholine (Fig. 63).

Evidence for the high sensitivity of the arterial wall to these physiologically active substances was given by the fact that under these conditions only a small proportion of the doses used had any action on the vessel walls. First, the internal carotid artery in the dog is relatively short (not exceeding about 70 mm) and wide (its lumen varies from 0.5 to 1.4 mm) and has no considerable bends (except the curvature in the cavernous sinus, whose wall occupies only 12% of the total surface area of the vessel). The blood flow in the artery must be predominantly laminar, so that only that portion of a substance flowing for about 10 sec in the peripheral layers of the blood or perfusion fluid could be in contact with the vessel walls, and most of it

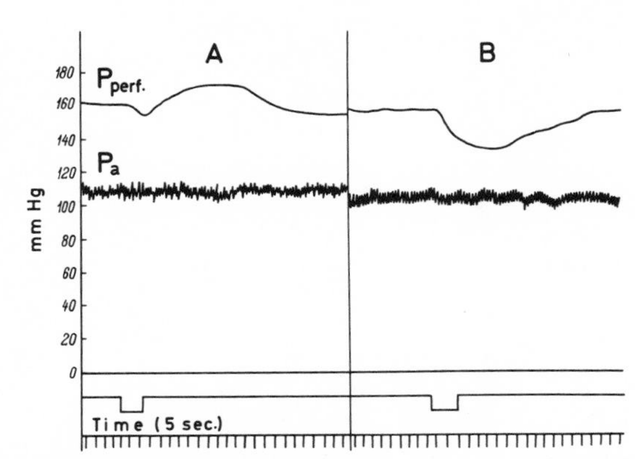

Fig. 63. Changes in resistance in the internal carotid artery of a dog, isolated *in situ*, in response to intra-arterial injection of 0.5 μg adrenalin (A) and to 0.5 μg acetylcholine (B) [257]. $P_{perf.}$, perfusion pressure in internal carotid artery; P_a, systemic arterial pressure. Marker shows time of injection of drugs.

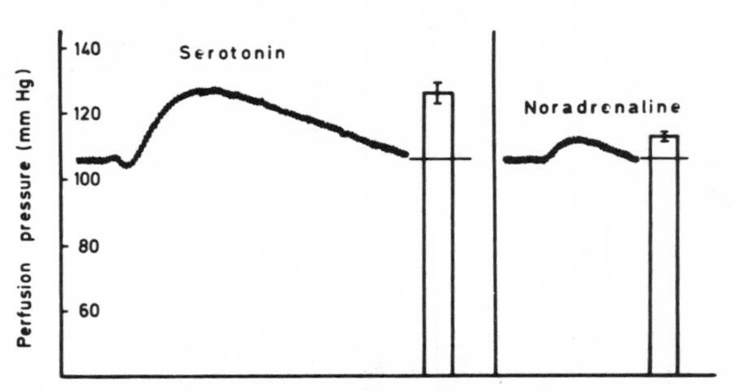

Fig. 64. Comparative magnitude of direct effects of equal doses of serotonin and noradrenalin on resistance of dog's internal carotid artery, isolated *in situ* and perfused with blood (see Chapter I for method). Columns show averaged values of effects with confidence limits [300].

would have no effect on them. Second, a certain proportion of any injected physiologically active substances must be rapidly destroyed by the appropriate blood enzymes (monoamine oxidase, cholinesterase, and so on).

Evidence for the specificity of the response of the internal carotid artery to cholinomimetic drugs was given by the strengthening of their effects after inhibition of cholinesterase by eserine (0.1-0.2 mg) and, in the case of adrenomimetics, after inhibition of monoamine oxidase by nialamide (1-2 mg). In both cases the effects of the corresponding mimetic agents were increased on the average by 30% compared with initially. On the other hand, the dilator effects produced by cholinomimetics of muscarine-like and nicotine-like action were considerably weakened after administration of the specific blocking agent, while the effects of α- and β-adrenomimetics as a rule were abolished by the corresponding α- and β-adrenergic blocking drugs [260].

The constrictor effects of serotonin were much greater than those of noradrenalin (Fig. 64), but the effect was limited to the major arteries of the brain [300] (Fig. 65). With an increase in the dose of serotonin, the magnitude of its effect rose exponentially, indicating gradual recruiting of more serotoninergic receptors in this process until no more were left "vacant" (Fig. 66),

Evidence for the specificity of action of serotonin is given by the fact that its vasoconstrictor action is greatly reduced or abolished altogether after injection of antiserotonin agents. Blockade of the tryptamine D receptors by ergotamine (0.2 mg), Hydergine (0.1 mg), and chlorpromazine (0.1 mg) abolishes (by 82-100%) the effects of serotonin. Blockade of the tryptamine M receptors by atropine (0.2 mg) and cocaine (0.2 mg) reduces the effect of serotonin by 37-40%. This evidently indicates that the walls of the internal carotid ar-

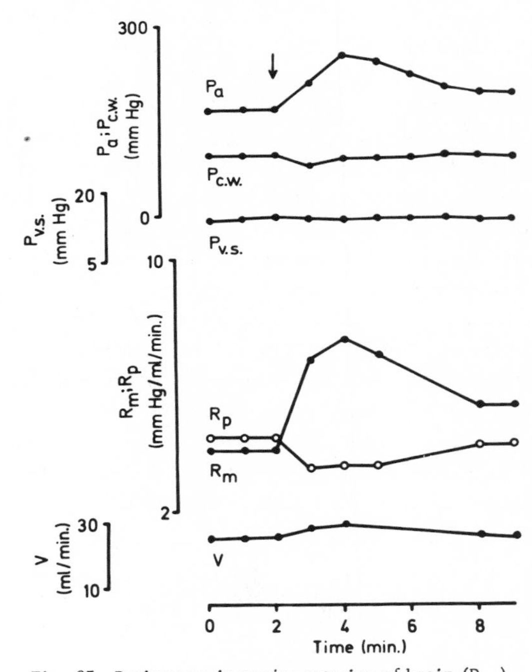

Fig. 65. Resistance in major arteries of brain (R_m) and in small arteries located peripherally to circle of Willis (R_p) calculated by means of a mathematical model from experimentally recorded perfusion pressure in internal carotid artery of dog isolated in situ (P_{perf}), and pressures in circle of Willis (P_{cW}) and in venous sinuses of brain following injection of serotonin (2 μg) into investigated internal carotid artery. Volume velocity of blood flow calculated from results obtained [248].

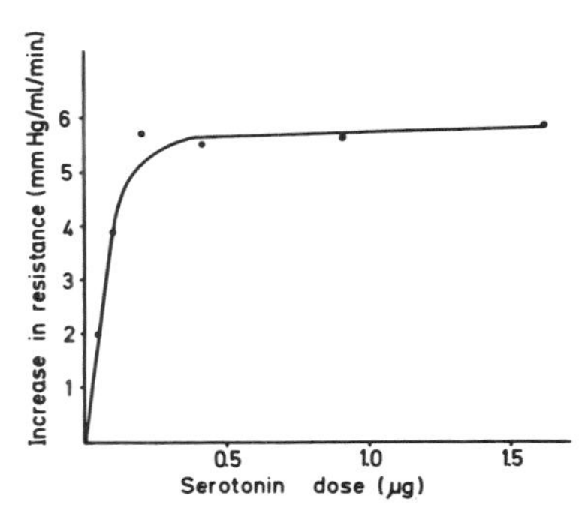

Fig. 66. Changes in resistance in internal carotid artery of dog, isolated in situ, as a function of dose of intra-arterially injected serotonin [258].

tery contain principally tryptamine D receptors [300].

Physiologically active substances circulating in the blood stream can thus exert a considerable effect on the walls of the internal carotid arteries, causing them to constrict or to dilate, and in this way they determine the functional behavior of these vessels under different conditions.

The absence of responses of the internal carotid arteries in dogs to the direct action of physiologically active substances, observed by some investigators after exclusion of all connections with the extracranial vessels [97], could be dependent either on the depth of anesthesia or on the animal's serious condition after the operation.

Sympathetic and Other Nervous Effects on the Major Arteries

Nerves running to the arteries of the brain and entering their walls have been studied since the end of last century. It has been shown that they are branches of autonomic (sympathetic, vagus, etc.) and somatic (especially cranial) nerves [388, 148, 175]. The major arteries of the brain are particularly richly innervated. The internal carotid plexus consists of bundles of medullated and nonmedullated nerve fibers, and contains nerve cells, both singly and in groups. Besides branches arising from the superior cervical sympathetic ganglion, this plexus also receives branches from the optic, occulomotor, trochlear, trigeminal, and abducent nerves [273, 312, 68]. Branches have also been described from the glossopharyngeal, vagus, and superior laryngeal nerves [175]. The nervous plexus of the vertebral arteries receives, besides sympathetic branches (from the inferior and middle cervical ganglia), branches from the vagus nerve and from the first to the eighth cervical spinal nerves [375].

The innervation of the human internal carotid arteries has recently been investigated in detail [30, 31] throughout their extent from the carotid sinus to the circle of Willis. The receptor apparatus is richly represented in the region of the carotid sinuses. Receptors of a rather different structure were also found in the cranial part of the vessel, especially in the region of the curvatures of the internal carotid artery. However, a rich efferent innervation is particularly characteristic of the intracavernous part of the artery: the adventitia contains a powerful plexus of bundles consisting of very thin, nonmedullated nerve fibers; a second plexus is present at the boundary between the adventitia and the media, from which thin fibrils penetrate into the depth of the muscular layer in which they form a third dense plexus.

The same author has recently studied the effector innervation of the internal carotid artery in dogs by histochemical methods for the detection of acetylcholine esterase and noradrenalin [245]. The results showed that this part of the artery contains principally large nerve trunks and smaller trunks given off by the plexus located in the adventitia of the carotid sinus and running along the vessel parallel to its axis (Fig. 67A). They run in both the superficial and deep layers of the adventitia of the artery. Many of these nerve bundles evidently pass straight through this region to supply segments of this artery located inside the bone and the cavernous sinus. Two powerful plexuses of nerve fibers, superficial and deep (Fig. 67C), are found in the region of the curvature and the cavernous portion of the internal carotid artery, in its adventitia, while at the boundary with the media there is a dense network of small loops, composed of thin, delicate fibers, some of which penetrate into the superficial layers of the media (Fig. 67B). These nerve plexuses also contain ganglionic nerve cells, frequently occurring as small groups of 3-6 cells (Fig. 67D). Their bodies are oval in shape and contain a large and more translucent vesicular nucleus. An abundant noradrenergic perivascular plexus has been demonstrated in the adventitia of the vertebral and basilar arteries of monkeys [81]; this plexus was markedly reduced or completely absent after repeated constriction of these vessels caused by direct chemical stimulation of their walls. The rich efferent innervation of the internal carotid artery is further evidence of the active role of this vessel as an effector in the regulation of the cerebral cir-

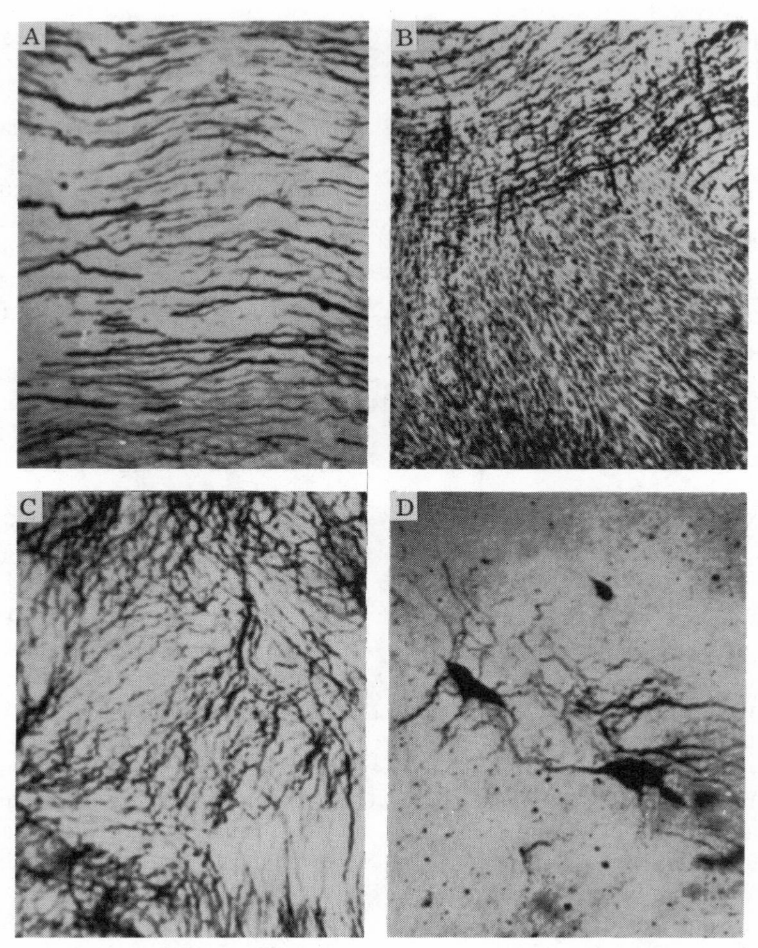

Fig. 67. Efferent innervation of different parts of the internal carotid artery in a dog (Koelle–Gomori method). A) periarterial plexus of nerve fibers containing cholinesterase in adventitia of cervical portion of vessel. Photomicrograph, 70X; B) Network of nerve fibers in surface layers of muscular coat in cavernous portion of artery. Photomicrograph, 90X; C) dense network of nerve fibers in deep layers of adventitia of cavernous portion of internal carotid artery. Photomicrograph, 100×; D) group of nerve cells containing active cholinesterase in adventitia of cavernous portion of vessel. Photomicrograph, 90X [245].

culation. The origin of nerve fibers discovered in walls of the major arteries of the brain has as yet received only little study. It has been shown [312] that many nonmedullated fibers in the nerve plexuses around the internal carotid arteries degenerate after removal of the ipsilateral superior cervical sympathetic ganglion; some fibers remain unchanged after this procedure and evidently have a different origin.

The presence of nervous control of the functional behavior of the major arteries of the brain might be concluded from the following experimental findings: although by direct electrical stimulation of the superior cervical sympathetic ganglia it was difficult to obtain clear constriction of the pial arteries, a decrease in the intensity of the cerebral circulation was observed by measuring the total blood flow in the brain by counting the drops of blood flowing from the sagittal sinus [116], by recording the perfusion pressure [26], by determining the velocity of the blood flow in the internal carotid artery [166], or by estimating the clearance of radioactive xenon in the brain [135]. However, this left unexplained the identity of the cerebral vessels on which the vasoconstrictor impulses act. The possibility is not ruled out that only the major arteries of the brain might receive these vasomotor influences, and as a result the intensity of the cerebral circulation is modified.

To solve this problem it was necessary to have special conditions under which the blood supply to the brain would not be disturbed during the investigation and the regulartory mechanisms would not prevent clear effects from being obtained. Thus it was best to carry out single experiments on the major arteries of the brain, for example, on one of the internal carotid arteries, for because of the existence of large anastomoses in the region of the circle of Willis, changes in the width of the lumen of this artery would have little, if any, effect on the blood supply to the brain. The effects of electrical stimulation of the ipsilateral superior cervical sympathetic ganglion on the internal carotid artery were studied [242, 243]. Changes in the lumen of these vessels were estimated by recording the blood flow in them by means of a photohemotachometer under the conditions indicated on page 8 in Chapter I.

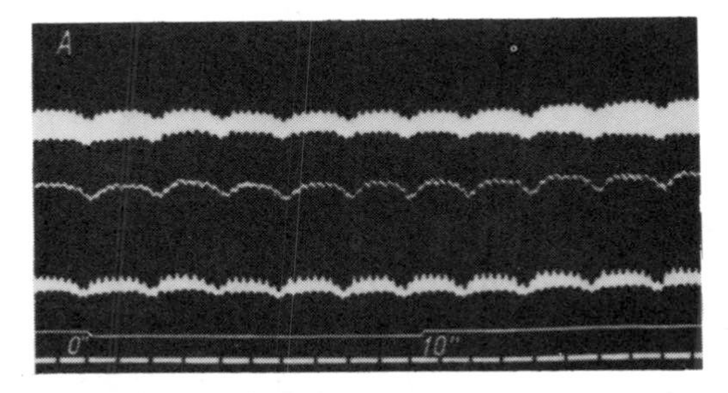

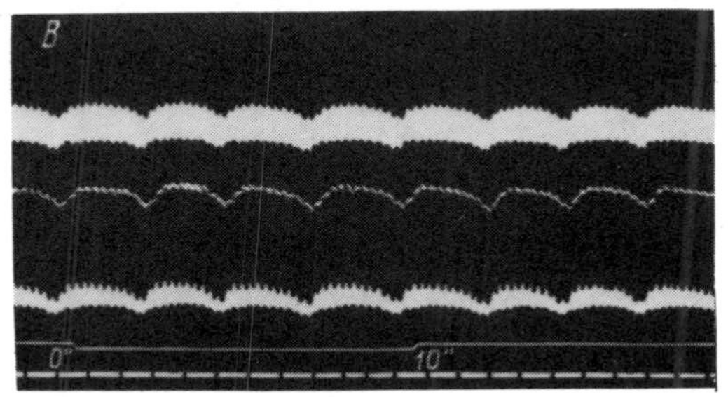

Fig. 68. Constriction of ipsilateral internal carotid artery in a dog during electrical stimulation of the superior cervical sympathetic ganglion with an intensity of 2 V (A). Absence of effect of stimulation (3 V) after intravenous injection of ergotamine in a dose of 0.1 mg/kg body weight (B) [242, 243]. From top to bottom: volume velocity of blood flow in internal carotid artery (on side of stimulation); systemic arterial pressure, 110 mm Hg (pressure compensator in action); volume velocity of blood flow in right (control) internal carotid artery; marker of stimulation; time marker (1 sec). Values of volume velocity of blood flow in left internal carotid artery for A: 0 sec, 1.27 ml/sec; 10 sec, 0.95 ml/sec; for B: for entire tracing 1.34 ml/sec.

In dogs the degree of constriction of the ipsilateral internal carotid artery (judging from the diminution of the blood flow) in response to electrical stimulation (2 V) ranged from 17 to 72% of its initial value in different experiments (Fig. 68), and during stronger stimulation (6 V) the blood flow usually stopped, indicating total occlusion of the lumen of the internal carotid artery. The absence of effect on the contralateral internal carotid artery suggested that neither the vessels of the circle of Willis nor segments of the cerebral vessels located peripherally to it changed their lumen. After intravenous injection of ergotamine (0.1 mg/kg body weight), stimulation of the cervical sympathetic ganglia did not reduce the blood flow in the internal carotid artery in dogs over a period of 15-30 min (Fig. 68).

The vasoconstrictor effect of the cervical sympathetic chain on the ipsilateral major arteries of the brain has also been demonstrated by other workers, although they usually did not interpret their results from the point of view of the nervous control of these large arteries. For instance, when a modified Rein's thermostromuhr was used to record the blood flow, a decrease in its intensity was found in the internal carotid arteries during stimulation of the superior cervical sympathetic ganglia, and in the vertebral arteries during stimulation of the stellate ganglia [356]. Similar results were obtained in experiments on dogs in which all anastomoses connecting the internal and external carotid arteries were preliminarily divided [380]. Further, in response to strong stimulation of the cervical sympathetic chain, the pressure in the basilar artery was lowered in cats, direct evidence of an increase in the resistance in the major arteries of the brain [363]. Following sympathetic stimulation, a decrease in the blood flow in the internal carotid artery, measured by an electromagnetic flowmeter, was also recently observed in monkeys [272].

Consequently, the experimental data indicate that the internal carotid arteries are under control of the sympathetic nervous system. However, this system seems not to be the only source of vasomotor innervation of the major arteries to the brain. Experiments to investigate reflex effects on these vessels from the baroreceptors of the venous sinuses of the brain showed that these effects persist even after total cervical sympathectomy, from the superior cervical ganglion to the stellate ganglion inclusive [254]. This indicated that some constrictor reflexes on the internal carotid and vertebral arteries may take place in the absence of the cervical sympathetic trunk. The existence of several different sources of innervation of the major arteries of the brain must have an important physiological significance, because if some nerve fibers were damaged, these vessels would not be denervated and thus deprived of their control by the nervous system.

The effects of stimulation of various nerves on resistance in the major arteries of the brain are reported in the literature, although when they describe the results of their experiments, writers frequently have not stated which parts of the vascular system of the brain reacted to such stimulation. For example, in response to stimulation of the vagus nerve, the pressure in the cirlce of Willis was observed to fall, and it did so to a greater degree and for longer than the systemic arterial pressure [407]; during stimulation of interoceptors of the spleen (increased congestion of the spleen with blood following ligation of the splenic veins or a decrease in the inflow of blood into the spleen after ligation of its artery), in some experiments a decrease in the pressure in the circle of Willis was observed, while the systemic arterial pressure remained unchanged [310]. In these experiments, therefore, the resistance in the major arteries of the brain seemed to be increased. In other experiments, during stimulation of the peroneal nerve, simultaneously with an increase in the blood flow in different parts of the brain (recorded by means of thermoelectrodes), the blood pressure in the circle of Willis increased while the systemic arterial pressure remained unchanged [156, 303]; in the writer's opinion this also must indicate a decrease in resistance in the major arteries of the brain resulting in an increase in the cerebral circulation. Finally, in experiments on dogs in which some parts of the floor of the fourth ventricle were stimulated, the blood pressure in the circle of Willis rose, while the systemic arterial pressure was unchanged [389]. This also indicated the lowering of resistance in the major arteries of the brain under these conditions.

Periodic fluctuations in the lumen of the internal carotid arteries were identified by simultaneous recordings of the intensity of the blood flow in both internal carotid arteries by means of flow-

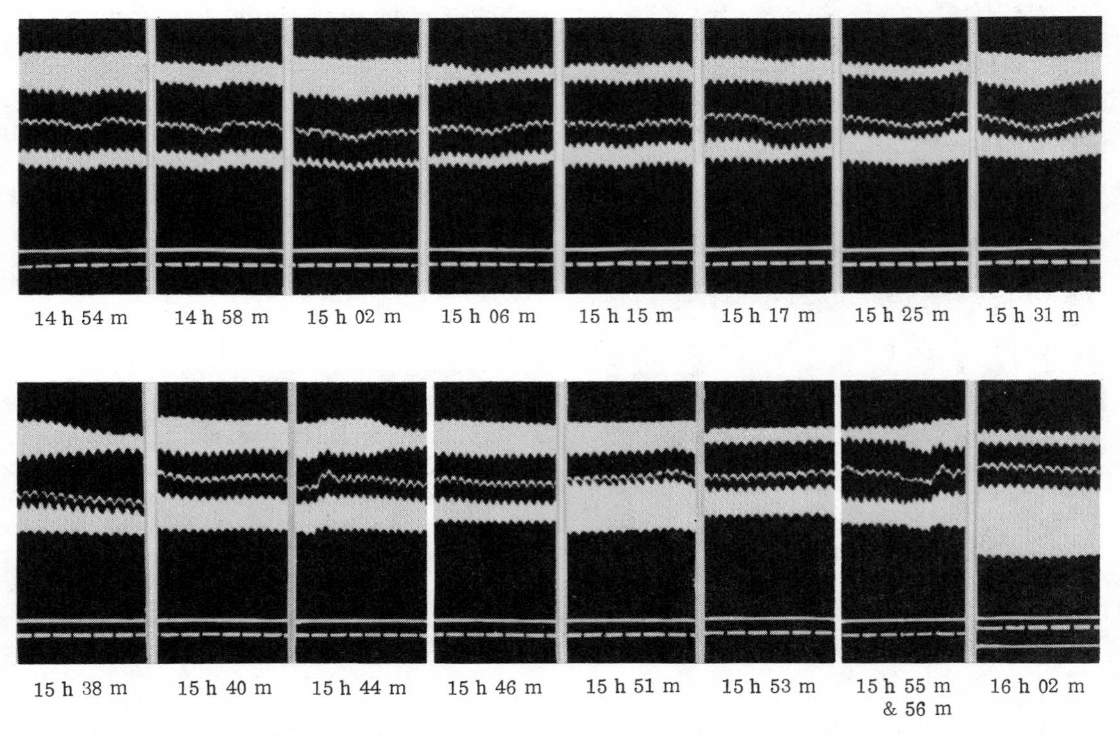

Fig. 69. Periodic changes of blood flow in the internal carotid arteries in a dog. Absolute values of volume velocity of blood flow are given in Table 7 [242, 243]. From top to bottom: volume velocity of blood flow in left internal carotid artery; general arterial pressure (125 mm Hg); volume velocity of blood flow in right internal carotid artery; time marker (1 sec). Numbers below tracings indicate time of recording. At 15 h 40 min arterial pressure was not increased, but pen was raised.

TABLE 7. Volume Velocities of Blood Flow in Left and Right Internal Carotid Arteries of a Dog in Experiment Illustrated in Fig. 69

Parameters measured	Time																
	14 h 54 min	14 h 58 min	15 h 02 min	15 h 06 min	15 h 15 min	15 h 17 min	15 h 25 min	15 h 31 min	15 h 38 min	15 h 40 min	15 h 44 min	15 h 46 min	15 h 51 min	15 h 53 min	15 h 55 min	15 h 56 min	16 h 02 min
Volume velocity of blood flow (ml/sec):																	
In left artery	0.93	0.64	0.93	0.64, 0.45	0.55	0.71	0.55	0.87	0.84, 0.55	0.84	0.87, 0.64	0.87	0.78	0.50	0.50	0.78	0.55
In right artery	0.55	0.55	0.00	0.39	0.64	0.64	0.74	0.64	0.71	0.81	0.81	0.59	1.01	0.71	0.71	0.84	1.25
General arterial pressure (mm Hg)	125	120	117	118	120	120	120	120	120	120	120	120	120	120	120	120	120

meters (Fig. 69 and Table 7). They were proved to be a manifestation of vasomotor control, for they were absent under deep anesthesia and they disappeared after intravenous injection of ergotamine (0.1 mg/kg body weight) [242, 243].

Role of Reflexes from the Carotid Sinus Receptors in Autoregulatory Responses of Major Arteries

It was shown in Chapter II that the major arteries of the brain play an important role both in damping relatively fast fluctuations (pulsatile and respiratory, for example) of the systemic arterial pressure and in regulating the constancy of the inflow of blood into the circle of Willis during relatively slow changes in the perfusion pressure of the brain. The major arteries of the brain thus seem to be responsible for the autoregulation of the cerebral circulation. The problem of the physiological mechanisms of these responses of the internal carotid and vertebral arteries must now be considered. Constriction of the major arteries of the brain during an increase in the systemic arterial pressure and their dilatation during its decrease could be, on the one hand, a component of a generalized vascular response modifying the level of the systemic arterial pressure or, on the other hand, they could be a manifestation of regulation of the inflow of blood into the brain. In the latter case they could be a myogenic response of the vessel wall to changes in the transmural pressure (a), i.e., a Bayliss effect, a hemodynamic effect of the properties of blood flow in the major arteries of the brain distinguished by the unique geometry of their lumen (the presence of curvatures, etc.),(b), or manifestations of the nervous control of the major arteries of the brain by reflexes from certain receptors (c). The results given below shed some light on this problem.

Constriction of the arteries of various organs, leading to an increase in the systemic peripheral resistance, is one possible cause of elevation of the systemic arterial pressure; dilatation of the arteries, on the other hand, lowers this pressure. In the cases described above the width of the internal carotid and vertebral arteries varied in the same direction as that of vessels in other parts of the body. However, the major arteries of the brain evidently do not participate as a component in the systemic vascular response producing changes in the arterial pressure. The following evidence supports this hypothesis: in cases when these arteries compensate for disturbances of the cerebral circulation, such as in traumatic edema or venous stagnation in the brain, the major arteries of the brain regularly constrict, whereas the systemic arterial pressure falls, i.e., when arteries in other parts of the body evidently dilate. Consequently, when the regulation of systemic arterial pressure requires dilatation of the internal carotid and vertebral arteries, and regulation of the blood supply to the brain, on the other hand, requires their constriction, these arteries actually are constricted. Hence it follows that these arteries are mainly concerned with regulation of the cerebral circulation. Furthermore, these results also give evidence against the view that constriction of the major arteries of the brain in response to elevation of the systemic arterial pressure is a myogenic Bayliss effect, for in traumatic edema and venous stagnation of the brain these arteries constrict simultaneously with a tendency for the systemic arterial pressure to fall; further supporting evidence is given by experiments in which constriction of the major arteries of the brain did not develop immediately, but only in response to the third or fourth elevation of the systemic arterial.

It can be concluded from these observations that constriction of the major arteries of the brain during elevation of the systemic arterial pressure, and their dilatation when the pressure falls can be regarded as manifestations of activity of the mechanism regulating a constant inflow of blood into the cerebrovascular system when the level of the systemic arterial pressure is changing. However, the physiological mechanisms responsible for this functional behavior of the system of the major arteries of the brain have hardly been studied.

This regulation could be neurogenic in character, although the location of the receptor areas for these reflexes and the parts of the central nervous system where their arcs are closed are unknown. It might be conjectured that the reflexes regulating the functional behavior of the major arteries of the brain could arise from the carotid receptors. In most experimental studies, however, stimulation of the baroreceptors was followed by reflex dilatation of the cerebral arteries. Ask-Upmark [6] showed that active dilatation of the pial arteries undoubtedly took place in response to electrical stimulation of the nerves from the carotid sinus, just as in response to an increase in pressure within the isolated carotid sinus in cats, and this dilatation was independent of a fall in the systemic arterial pressure (it appeared sooner and also occurred in experiments in which the pressure was stabilized). This indicated the existence of a vasodilator reflex from the carotid sinus baroreceptors to the blood vessels of the brain. The existence of similar reflex dilatation of the cerebral blood vessels has subsequently been confirmed by other workers [338, 24, 25, 334, 335, 307, 277], although in their experiments the conditions were very complicated and it was difficult, therefore, to obtain conclusive evidence for reflex influences from the carotid baroreceptors on the cerebral circulation. Which of the cerebral blood vessels are to be considered as effectors of the vasomotor reflexes from the carotid sinus receptors to the brain circulation is another problem that did not engage the attention of the researchers cited.

It might be supposed that reflex effects from the carotid sinus receptors on the cerebral circulation are brought about, at least partly, through the major arteries of the brain. This problem has been studied by the author and his associates in dogs with an isolated carotid sinus [85]. The behavior of the internal carotid arteries was assessed from quantitative measurements of the volume velocity of the blood flow in these vessels (see Chapter I). To exclude any effect of changes in the systemic arterial pressure, where necessary, this was stabilized. During perfusion of the isolated carotid sinus with Ringer solution the blood flow in the internal carotid artery could remain stable for a long time. However, as soon as physiologically active substances (adrenalin, noradrenalin, acetylcholine, etc.) were added to the perfusion fluid, the volume velocity of the blood flow was immediately changed in the ipsilateral (and in some cases, the contralateral) internal carotid artery (Fig. 70); if the carotid sinus was denervated, these effects disappeared. The values of the reflex changes in volume velocity of blood flow in the ipsilateral internal carotid arteries produced in these experiments while the arterial pressure remained stable, were as follows (the initial blood flow was taken as 100%): adrenalin (0.5 mg during 10 sec)* – 62 – 9%, and acetylcholine (0.5 mg during 10 sec)* – 211 – 30%. Even when the blood flow in the internal carotid arteries remained stable during stimulation of the carotid sinus receptors, the responses of their walls to small doses

* The necessity of using relatively large doses of these substances is evidently explained by the reduced sensitivity of the receptors when deprived of their normal blood supply throughout the period of the experiment, by the possible damage to some of the nerve fibers during the operation to isolate the carotid sinus, and by the usually deep anesthesia under which the animals took part in the acute experiments.

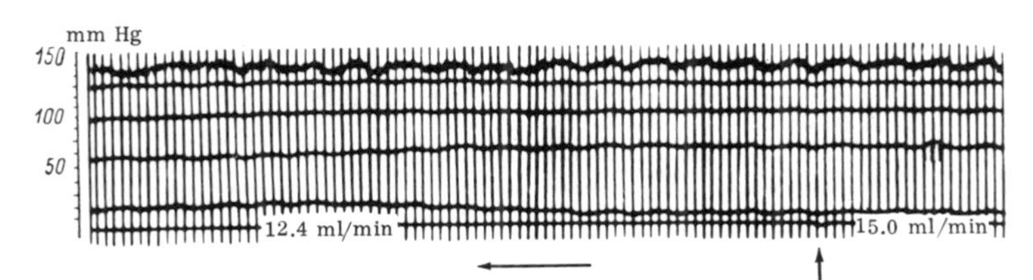

Fig. 70. Reflex effects from carotid sinus chemoreceptors on ipsilateral internal carotid arteries in a dog: constriction of ipsilateral internal carotid artery after addition of adrenalin (0.5 mg) over a 10-sec period to perfusion fluid of the isolated carotid sinus [85]. From top to bottom: systemic arterial pressure (scale on left), two levels of differential carotid artery; the same in the right (ipsilateral) internal carotid artery; volume velocities indicated below curves. Arrows denote beginning of injection of substances into the sinus. Vertical lines are time markers (1 sec). Curves to be read from right to left.

(0.1-2.0 μg) of physiologically active substances (adrenalin, acetylcholine, etc.) injected intra-arterially were regularly altered. Both the threshold of the response (the artery reacted to smaller or larger doses of the substance) and the magnitude of the effect, which was increased or decreased were altered. Thus, after addition of adrenalin to the perfusion fluid of the isolated carotid sinus, the local constrictor effect of the same substance increased on the average by 23%, while after addition of acetylcholine the direct dilator effect on the internal carotid artery increased by an average of 116%.

The possible physiological significance of these reflex effects from the carotid sinus chemoreceptors on the ipsilateral internal carotid arteries must next be considered, remembering that the same stimuli may have identical effects when acting directly on the vessel wall. First, the specialized carotid sinus chemoreceptors may evidently be more sensitive to many factors than the walls of the internal carotid arteries themselves; second, if constriction or dilatation of the internal carotid arteries takes place through a reflex mechanism, it can be coordinated in the central nervous system with other responses of the vascular system participating in regulation of the cerebral circulation.

Reflex Vasoconstriction Arising from Intracranial Receptors

It might be supposed that the constriction of the major arteries of the brain taking place in traumatic cerebral edema develops by a reflex mechanism, since the active segments of these arteries are located extracranially and their mechanical compression was therefore ruled out. However, the role of intracranial baroreceptors (whose function is described in [327]) was excluded because constriction of the major arteries of the brain in the present experiments was also observed after extensive trephining of the skull. A role of dural mechanoreceptors (reflex effects of which on the systemic arterial pressure have been observed elsewhere [23, 395]) can likewise be excluded, first, because constriction of the major arteries of the brain in edema was also observed after extensive opening of the dura, and second, because strong electrical stimulation of the dura, in the present author's experiments, like mechanical stretching, did not affect the pressure gradient along the length of the major arteries of the brain, i.e., was not reflected in their resistance. It could further be suggested that reflex constriction of the internal carotid and vertebral arteries arises as a result of stimulation of the pial mechanoreceptors following an increase in brain volume during the time of edema [228]. However, the existence of such a reflex has not yet been revealed in physiological experiments. Hence, although reflex constriction of the major arteries of the brain during manifest edema is apparently the most probable mechanism of this vascular reaction, the receptive zone of the reflex and its pathways are still unexplained.

After it had been found that the occlusion of the jugular veins is followed by constriction of the major arteries of the brain, an attempt was made to elucidate the physiological mechanism responsible for this above mentioned vasoconstrictor response [209]. Experiments showed that an important condition for obtaining this effect is sudden and simultaneous occlusion of all jugular veins, and not their consecutive occlusion, i.e., an increase in the blood pressure (even though only temporary) in the venous system of the brain is undoubtedly essential. Next, if Ringer's solution was injected rapidly through one of the external jugular veins in a cranial direction, the same effect as that of occlusion of all the jugular veins was sometimes obtained. If the effect did not arise, the probable reason was that the pressure in the venous system of the skull could not be made to rise, possibly because of well-developed collateral communications with the opposite jugular vein. In fact, when the second jugular vein was also occluded (the effect of successive occlusion of the jugular veins was usually slight), a sudden reduction in the inflow of blood into the circle of Willis took place.

It could be postulated, on the basis of these experiments, that constriction of the major arteries of the brain under these conditions takes place through a reflex from the baroreceptors of the venous sinuses of the brain [215, 254]. In further experiments the baroreceptors of the venous sinuses of the rabbit's brain were stimulated by injecting fluid (Ringer's solution, dextran, or blood), warmed to body temperature, into them under pressure. All branches of the external jugular veins except the temporal emissary veins, connecting them directly to the transverse sinuses of the brain, were first carefully ligated (see Chapter I). Liquid was infused into the transverse sinuses through a polyethylene catheter tied into the jugular vein in a cranial direction; a similar catheter on the contralateral side enabled changes taking place under these conditions in the venous pressure in the brain sinuses to be recorded. A third polyethylene catheter, introduced through the external jugular vein as far as the cranial vena cava, was used to record the blood pressure in the latter vessels. During infusion of fluid into the transverse sinus, it appeared to be difficult to raise the pressure throughout the venous system of the brain, despite the fact that in these experiments the external jugular veins were occluded on both sides, (in rabbits, these veins play an important role in the drainage of blood from the brain); this result can evidently be explained by the well-developed collateral outflow of blood through the venous system of the spine. However, when a relatively large volume of fluid was injected, the venous pressure in the contralateral transverse sinus rose slightly (by 0.5-3.5 cm water). Simultaneously, the blood pressure in the circle of Willis fell, whereas the systemic arterial pressure either underwent a transient decrease or remained stable (when the experiments were carried out on the thorax–head preparation; see Chapter I). Since the resistance in the vascular system of the brain peripheral to the circle of Willis was increased at this time through constriction of the pial arteries, and also through the artificial raising of the venous pressure, it can be concluded that the increase in pressure difference along the course of the major arteries of the brain is evidence of their constriction. So

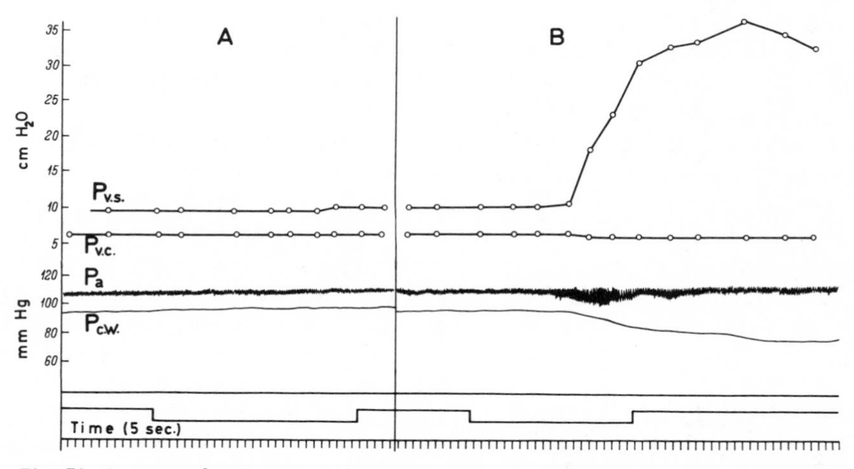

Fig. 71. Increase of resistance in the major arteries of the brain during elevation of the pressure in the venous sinuses following infusion of liquid into them. Experiment on thorax–head preparation [254]. $P_{v.s.}$, venous pressure in transverse sinus; $P_{v.c.}$, venous pressure in cranial vena cava (pressure compensator connected to that vessel); P_a, arterial pressure in aorta: $P_{c.W.}$, arterial pressure in circle of Willis. Marker shows period of infusion of fluid into transverse sinus (A 0.23 ml/sec and B 0.32 ml/sec).

long as the venous pressure in the sinuses of the brain remained unincreased, the pressure difference in the aorta and in the circle of Willis was unchanged (Fig. 71A), but as soon as it began to rise, the pressure difference immediately started to increase (Fig. 71B).

A rich system of receptors have been found morphologically in the walls of the venous sinuses of the brain, especially the cavernous sinus [196, 274]. The following experimental data have demonstrated the functions of receptors of this type: if the pressure in the sagittal [394] and in the cavernous [275] sinuses rises, a reflex decrease in the systemic arterial pressure takes place. It may naturally be suggested that the effects on the major arteries of the brain referred to above also were produced by reflexes from the baroreceptors of the venous sinuses. However, it was first necessary to rule out purely mechanical compression of the major arteries of the brain through an increase in pressure in the venous sinuses, as occurred in experiments on cadavers [371]. Evidence against such a possibility was obtained in the author's experiments: first, the degree of elevation of the venous pressure in the present experiments was small, usually not more than 2.5-3.5 cm water, and this could not have produced any appreciable compression of the arteries; second, the elevation of pressure in the brain sinuses and the degree of constriction of the major arteries of the brain were not completely parallel, i.e., they took place about at the same time, but usually constriction of the internal carotid and vertebral arteries continued for some time after termination of the infusion and the fall in venous pressure. It can therefore be concluded that reflex constriction of the major arteries of the brain takes place in response to an increase in blood pressure in the system of venous sinuses of the brain [216, 254]. This reflex vasoconstriction was observed during stimulation of the baroreceptors of the intracranial venous system, but when in control experiments the pressure in the extracranial veins of the head was increased, this reaction of the major arteries of the brain did not take place. The systemic arterial pressure was usually raised in such cases, whereas it regularly fell in response to stimulation of the baroreceptors of the brain sinuses. The nervous pathways of this reflex from the venous sinuses of the brain on its major arteries are not yet known. Bilateral extirpation of the superior and inferior (stellate) cervical sympathetic ganglia and of the lateral trunk (in experiments on rabbits) did not abolish this effect. Consequently, this reflex takes place (either always or only after sympathectomy) without involvement of the efferent pathways of the cervical sympathetic chain.

The reflex constriction of the major arteries of the brain in response to an increase of pressure in its venous sinuses, described above, is a special case of the "veno-vasomotor" reflexes [390, 190]. This reflex protects the brain, as it lies in the rigid skull, against overfilling of its vessels with blood should the venous drainage be disturbed.

CHAPTER VII

THE PIAL ARTERIES

As was shown above, it is the pial arteries (especially the small ones) which play an important role in regulating the adequate blood supply to the brain tissue in order to meet its metabolic requirements. These arteries dilate when the neural elements experience a deficient blood supply, especially if the existing blood supply is inadequate at a time when activity is considerably increased. Under these conditions, influences from the brain tissues on the arteries supplying them with blood (i.e., feedback) can take place either by direct action of vasodilator metabolites accumulating in the blood vessel walls, or by the intervention of vasomotor nervous impulses, not necessarily involving the participation of the vasomotor center of the medulla, which is known to be obligatorily concerned only in regulating the level of the systemic arterial pressure.

Humoral Feedback from the Brain Tissue to the Pial Arteries

Ever since the 1950s the view has been widely held that the increase in blood supply to the tissues of the brain, when their metabolic demands are increased, depends on the direct action of vasodilator metabolites on the vessel walls. A particularly important role has been ascribed to carbon dioxide [344, 170, 198, 364, 142, 405, 200] which, besides being an end-product of metabolism, is also a powerful vasodilator of the cerebral vessels – in fact, the most powerful known at that time. It was therefore commonly supposed that the CO_2 which accumulates in the brain tissue every time the blood supply is deficient [266] diffuses to the walls of the small cerebral and pial arteries and causes them to dilate. The main experimental results relating to this problem are as follows [264, 266]: stopping the artificial respiration, the addition of carbon dioxide to the inspired air, and acidosis resulting from intravenous injection of acids were accompanied by an increase in the CO_2 concentration detected on the brain surface by selective electrodes, and by an increase in the blood flow in the cortex recorded by means of thermistors. In experiments in which, on the other hand, the CO_2 tension in the blood was reduced (hyperventilation, hypoglycemia, alkalosis following intravenous injection of alkalies), a decrease in the blood flow to the brain was observed. However, these results did not prove the role of CO_2 in the genesis of functional hyperemia in the brain, because in all the experiments described above the CO_2 concentration increased primarily in the blood, and the CO_2 could act directly on the cerebral vessels, causing them to dilate; the substance THAM, which binds the carbon dioxide of the blood, accordingly abolished the vasodilatation. Conversely, in Meyer's experiments acetazolamide ("diamox"), a carbonic anhydrase inhibitor, prevented the removal of CO_2 from the tissues, so that when this inhibitor was given by intravenous injection, the quantity of carbon dioxide in the brain tissues rose sharply, yet the circulation in the brain was not increased; Meyer explained this result by assuming that acetazolamide prevents the formation of H^+ and HCO_3^-, and thus abolishes the action of CO_2 on the vessel walls. Later, other workers [200] observed that acetazolamide abolishes the increased blood flow in the visual cortex during photic stimulation.

The dilator effect of an increase in the carbon dioxide concentration in the blood on the blood vessels of the brain has frequently been studied [224, 105], and this effect has been shown to take place even in the intrauterine period [197]. It is abolished or distorted in ischemia of the cerebral cortex [399]. As a result of investigations of the quantitative relationship between the increased blood flow in the brain and the CO_2 concentration in the blood, some workers have concluded that the decrease in cerebrovascular resistance under these conditions depends less on the direct effect of CO_2 on the walls of the resistive arteries, and more on the resulting changes in pH of the extracellular brain fluid [19, 20, 21, 350]. However, in this case also the correlation between the intensity of the blood flow and changes in pH was not very high

[203]. It is accordingly open to question whether changes in the CO_2 tension or changes in pH in the extracellular brain fluid can act as the direct mediator of vasodilator stimuli to the brain vessels. These doubts are strengthened still further by the fact, cited in [351], that during perfusion of an isolated cerebral artery with blood containing different concentrations of CO_2, no corresponding changes in the resistance to the blood flow were found.

On the other hand, the results of some experiments indicate that the dilator action of CO_2 in the brain may involve the participation of neurogenic mechanisms. For instance, dihydroergotamine abolishes the increased blood flow from the sagittal sinus produced in cats [127] by inhalation of a gas mixture containing a high CO_2 concentration. Other experiments [41, 167, 166] have shown that in dogs, inhalation of a gas mixture containing 15-40% CO_2 causes vasodilatation accompanied by signs of desynchronization visible in the electrocorticogram; barbiturates, influencing electrical activity alone, weakened the vasodilator effect of CO_2. Further work has shown that the dilator effect of CO_2 on the cerebral blood vessels may be brought about by a reflex from chemoreceptors situated either in the venous sinuses [336] or elsewhere around the subarachnoid space [252, 253]. Evidence for the role of the vasomotor center in the effect of carbon dioxide on the cerebral circulation has also been obtained [277].

The following experimental data are against the role of CO_2 as the chief feedback mechanism responsible for functional hyperemia in the brain. Spontaneous fluctuations in the intensity of the cortical circulation were found in cats during steady breathing, and in the opinion of the investigators concerned [136], this is more likely to be explained by the influence of the autonomic innervation on the vessels than by the action of CO_2 on them. Furthermore, in preparations of the isolated cat's cortex, the increase in blood flow accompanying bursts of electrical activity was completely independent of the CO_2 concentration in the blood [362]. Finally, it was found that a linear relationship exists in cats between the frequency index of the electroencephalogram and the local blood flow in the cortex, which was unaffected by differences in the CO_2 concentration in the blood of the experimental animals [122]. If carbon dioxide were in fact the principal transmitter of information to the cerebral vessels at a time of intensified activity of the brain neurons, its concentration in the blood would be found to be reflected in the relationship between the cortical blood flow and the level of its activity.

Since an adequate blood supply to the brain tissue is regulated in accordance with its metabolic demands, a question of particular interest arises: can the carbon dioxide formed in brain tissue diffuse into the region of the walls of the pial arteries in a quantity sufficient to cause them to dilate, thereby increasing the inflow of blood into the brain tissue. Carbon dioxide possesses a high coefficient of diffusion [358], and it can therefore diffuse rapidly through the tissue membranes to reach the pial arteries. A humoral action on the arteries by any other pathway cannot be contemplated because normally CO_2 only enters the capillaries and is carried away by the blood into the veins, and then into the lungs. In an actual case, when cortical activity was increased (the "recruiting response"), the CO_2 concentration in the outflowing blood was increased by 2-11 mm Hg, although this did not occur in all experiments [121]. With the onset of paroxysmal activity in the cortex following intravenous injection of metrazol, an increase in the CO_2 tension from 28 to 34 mm Hg, i.e., by 6 mm, was observed 30-40 sec later on the brain surface (in the region of the pial arteries [126].* However, it is not yet known whether this concentration of CO_2 could cause such marked vasodilatation of the pial arteries. This problem still remains unsolved today. An increase in the circulation in the cortex was observed when the CO_2 concentration in fluid irrigating the brain surface rises from 0 to 35% [95], i.e., by 266 mm Hg. Later this problem was studied in more detail [291]. When the CO_2 concentration in the medium surrounding the pial arteries was increased (to 5-10%, i.e., to 35-70 mm Hg), vasodilatation occurred in only half of the experiments, while in the rest vasoconstriction was observed or there was no effect. When a vasodilator effect was produced it seemed to be dependent on the direct action of carbon dioxide on the vessel walls and not on increased acidity of the medium, because vasodilatation was also observed in cases when the pH of the medium was unchanged. Dilatation of pial arteries of smaller caliber was more marked than in the case of larger vessels.

In a recent study [398] the direct effect of the pH of an artificial cerebrospinal fluid on the pial arteries of cats and rats was investigated by a micropipet technique. The weakly acid fluid A caused inconstant vasodilatation, while the strongly acid fluid B caused dilatation of the pial arteries in all

*No other quantitative data pertaining to the increase in CO_2 concentration in the extracellular fluid of the brain tissue during intensification of cerebral activity could be found in the literature.

experiments. However, it must be noted that the acidity of the solutions tested was far outside the physiological range: the pH of A was 5.48 ± 0.01 and of B 2.12 ± 0.01.* There is thus no substantial evidence to suggest that the direct effect of either the CO_2 or the acid pH of the extracellular fluid on the cerebral arterial walls plays a dominant role in the genesis of the functional hyperemia in the cerebral cortex under normal conditions.

Recently an attempt was made to analyze the mechanismis of dilatation of the pial arteries in rabbits brought about by a decrease in blood supply to the cerebral cortex (resulting from a stepwise drop of the systemic arterial pressure) [253]. From the point of view of the physiological mechanism of this vasodilatation, two problems require elucidation: first, what is the trigger mechanism for dilatation of the pial arteries and, second, how do the vasodilator stimuli reach the arterial walls? In previous studies, by analogy with responses of the smooth-muscle layers of hollow organs (in which contraction of the smooth muscles takes place in response to their stretching, and relaxation in response to decreased stretching), the reaction of vessel walls of that kind was described as the Bayliss effect [15, 78, 155]. Since this response of the vessel walls in the brain, as in other organs, persists after denervation or during the action of drugs blocking nervous conduction [75, 79, 314], the view became widely adopted that this phenomenon is myogenic in nature [63].

However, the following experimental facts obtained by the present writer [353] are against this hypothesis: a) with a fall of systemic arterial pressure, the intravascular pressure should have fallen more in the large pial arteries than in the small; in fact the small arteries dilated much sooner and to a greater degree than the large (see Fig. 12 in Chapter II); B) dilatation of the pial arteries was observed only 2 min 20 sec (small arteries) and 3 min 34 sec (large arteries) after lowering of the systemic arterial pressure; any direct relationship of cause and effect between these two findings is thus very doubtful. Another possible mechanism for dilatation of the pial arteries could be a primary decrease in the blood supply to the brain which, in turn, would influence the pial arteries. Such a relationship was highly probable, for they always dilated after a decrease in the local blood flow and after a decrease in pO_2 in the cerebral cortex. So far as the nature of the vasodilator stimuli, i.e., the mechanism of the feedback responsible for dilatation of the pial arteries, is concerned, a direct vasodilator effect of hypoxia on the cerebral vessels [265, 20] could be accepted because, in these experiments, a decrease in pO_2 in the brain always preceded dilatation of the pial arteries. However, a decrease in pO_2 in the brain tissues would not necessarily imply the direct action of hypoxia on the vessel walls. In fact, in the experiment concerned [253], dilatation of the pial arteries could not depend on the direct action of hypoxia on their walls, for pO_2 in the arterial blood (which is in the closest contact with the smooth-muscle cells of the small arteries) not only was not reduced, but was actually increased. So far as the vasodilator action of acid metabolic products (CO_2 or lactic acid, for exam-

*In the present author's experiments on dogs, even during very severe cerebral ischemia preceding death the pH of the extracellular fluid on the brain surface never fell below 6.0.

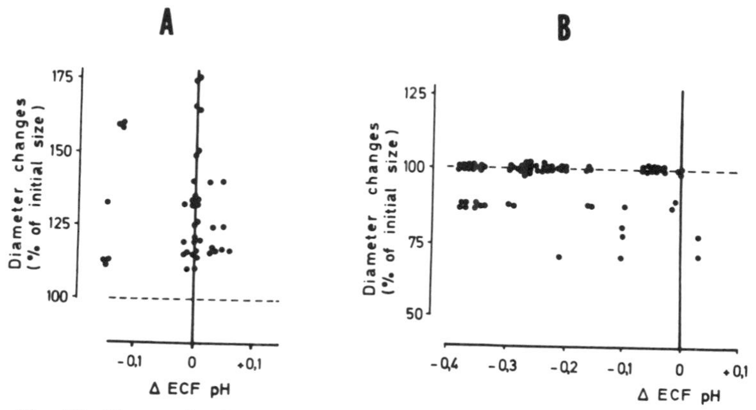

Fig. 72. Changes in pH in extracellular fluid of the cerebral cortex ECF with a decrease in systemic arterial pressure in rabbits on the average from 100 to 40 mm Hg in two series of experiments: in the presence (A) and absence (B) of autoregulatory dilatation of pial arteries [253]. Explanation in text.

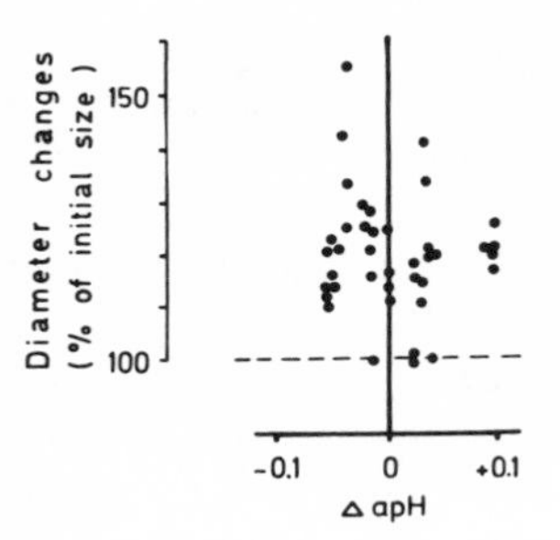

Fig. 73. Changes in pH of arterial blood with a decrease in systemic arterial pressure in rabbits of the average from 100 to 40 mm Hg at moments preceding autoregulatory dilatation of pial arteries [253].

ple, on the pial arteries is concerned, direct measurements of pH in the brain and in the arterial blood have not demonstrated any regular shift toward the acid side (Figs. 72A and 73). Consequently, there could be no direct relationship of cause and effect between dilatation of the pial arteries and the action of acid metabolites on their walls. Conversely, in the absence of compensatory dilatation of the pial arteries, in some experiments the pH of the brain was regularly shifted towards the acid side, but this did not give rise to vasodilatation (Fig. 72B). Dilatation of the pial arteries could not have been caused by the direct action of CO_2 for the additional reason that pCO_2 in the brain tissue was reduced, as is generally the case in hypoxia [19] as the result of compensatory hyperventilation. The only possible suggestion was, therefore, that the transmission of stimuli from the cerebral cortex, when subjected to a deficient blood supply and to hypoxia, to the pial arteries takes place by a neural route.

Nervous Feedback Mechanism from the Brain Tissue to the Pial Arteries

Under the light microscope both medullated and nonmedullated nerve fibers have been found in the walls of the pial as well as of the intracerebral arteries. They are a continuation of the nervous plexuses of the large arteries at the base of the brain and they extend along the vessels as far as the terminal branches of the arterioles. Nerve fibers were found on the surface of the adventitia of the arteries and deep inside their walls, at the boundary between the connective-tissue and muscular layers of the vessel walls [130, 117, 119, 273, 64, 175, 410, etc.]. Nerve fibers are particularly numerous in the region of branching of the cerebral arteries or where lateral branches divide from the main trunks [55]. Besides nerve fibers, unipolar cells of different sizes and shapes have been found in the walls of the pial arteries, and their processes ramify in the region of the walls of these vessels and among the connective tissue cells of the pia mater [1, 175]. On the basis of the morphological features, some workers have concluded that nerve fibers in the walls of the cerebral vessels may differ in nature. For instance, the thin, nonmedullated fibers which are found at the boundary between the adventitia and media of the vessels, and which give off small branches to the muscular layer, have been regarded as vasomotor fibers, while the medullated fibers on the surface of the adventitia of the vessels have been regarded as sensory [192, 128]. Less was known regarding the origin of nerve fibers in the region of the pial arteries. The absence of their degeneration after removal of the cervical sympathetic ganglia was initially explained by the origin of these nerve fibers from ganglion cells located along the course of the cerebral vessels [43, 306]. However, in later investigations, 18-20 days after cervical sympathectomy, degenerated nerve fibers were found in the region of the walls of the pial arteries [65]. Similar findings have been obtained with regard to individual nerve fibers in the choroid plexuses [387]. This indicates that the superior cervical sympathetic ganglia are evidently one of the sources of the vasomotor innervation of the cerebral arteries. In addition, nerve fibers, becoming medullated at an early stage arising from the oculomotor nerve and regarded as preganglionic [148], have also been described on the cerebral vessels.

Nervous structures which are usually regarded as receptors have also been found in the walls of the cerebral vessels. They are both simple and arborizing in type. Most of them lie in the adventitia of the vessels and in the surrounding connective tissue of the pia-arachnoid [103, 173, 128, 1]. Receptors have been found in the region of arteries and veins of different caliber, but they are most numerous on large arteries and veins [194, 274].

Nerve cells and fibers have thus been found in the walls of the blood vessels of the brain by many investigators who used classical histological techniques. The nature of these neural structures, however, has been studied only in recent years. By means of a histochemical technique demonstrating catecholamines in nerve structures, nerve fibers, giving a deep green fluorescence characteristic of catecholamines, were discovered in the region of the walls of the pial arteries of rabbits [67, 301]. These fibers frequently form thin bundles, each consisting of several fibers with numerous connections between them (Fig. 74A). A network of adrenergic nerve fibers thus exists in the adventitia of the pial vessels. They continue along the radial arteries which penetrate into the interior

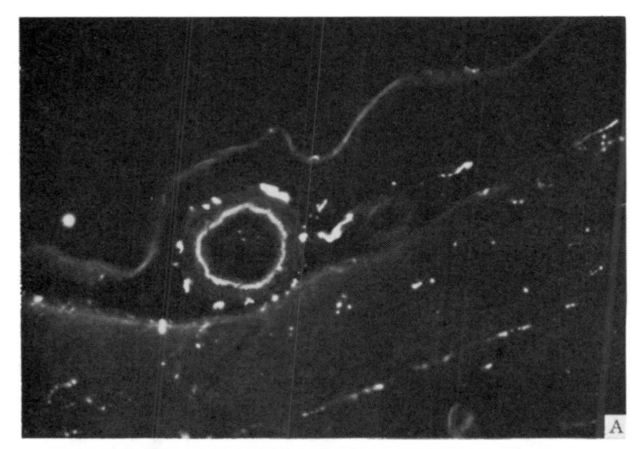

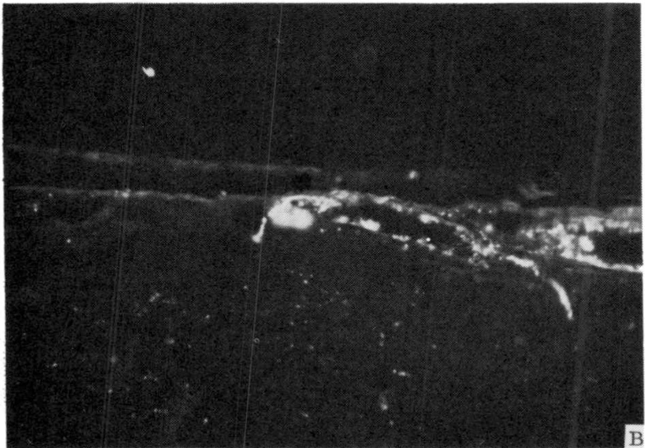

Fig. 74. Adrenergic nerve fibers in the walls of pial arteries and their collaterals to the pia mater and cerebral cortex in a rabbit [301]. A) Fluorescent neural structures in adventitia of pial artery divided transversely. They are also visible in the pia to the right of the artery. Internal elastic membrane of artery shows strong autofluorescence (present even without histochemical staining of the tissue). Arachnoid visible above vessels. Beneath them is the cortex where fluorescent nerve fibers are also visible. 310X. B) Two fluorescent nerve fibers leave the pial artery (divided obliquely) and enter the cortex. On left: nerve fiber, apparently accompanying radial artery; on right: fiber enters superficial layers of cortex independently of blood vessels; its course is oblique relative to the brain surface. 280X.

of the cortex. The neural bundles of the pial arteries give off nerve fibers, also with a green fluorescence, which run directly into the surface layer of the cortex (Fig. 74B). A study of serial sections showed that these cannot be the fibers accompanying the radial arteries; they differ from the latter in entering the cortex frequently at an acute angle to its surface. In total pial preparations a network of varicose fibers with green fluorescence can be seen: many of these, in the form of single fibers or thin bundles, represent nervous connections between the pial vessels. The nerve fibers of the pial arteries thus give off two types of collaterals which lose their connection with the vessel walls: some of these collaterals run into the cortex, while others enter the pia mater. Bilateral cervical sympathectomy caused the total disappearance of fluorescent nerve fibers in the region of the pial arteries and of the collaterals supplied by them to the pia and cortex, but the network of fluorescent fibers in the interior of the cortex remained. This showed that the nerve fibers belonging to the pial vessels are postsynaptic axons of the sympathetic nervous system. Pharmacological analysis showed that these nerve fibers near the walls of the pial arteries are adrenergic fibers containing noradrenalin [154]. The presence of adrenergic fibers, connecting the arteries with the superficial layers of the cortex, suggests that the connection between the cortex and these vessels may be closed also without the participation of the bulbar or any other vasomotor center. However, the extent to which these adrenergic fibers participate in functional dilatation of the pial arteries under natural condition has not yet been established. An adrenergic nervous plexus all along the pial arterial ramifications has also been demonstrated in cats [290] and rats [131].

Other histochemical investigations [174, 311] have shown in cats, rabbits, and rats the existence of numerous nerve fibers in the region of the walls of the pial arteries, containing active cholinesterase (and presumably, cholinergic). The greater the caliber of the arteries, the denser the interweaving of these fibers (Fig. 75A and B). Vessels of 100-200 and more μ in diameter contain both longitudinal and transverse fibers (Fig. 62A), while the smaller pial arteries are accompanied mainly by longitudinal cholinergic fibers. In general, such nerve fibers can be found in the region of pial arteries of all sizes, down to their smallest branches. The comparatively large arteries have a well-developed superficial (adventitial) plexus whose branches penetrate the vascular wall and form another plexus of thin nerve bundles within it, between the media and adventitia. In thick transverse sections containing a pial artery, running longitudinally, with the cortex lying beneath it, in some cases numerous cholinergic fibers connecting the cortex directly with the periarterial nerve plexus can be clearly seen (Fig. 75C). The direction of these nerve fibers is not yet clear: they run either from the periarterial vascular plexus into the cerebral cortex or vice versa.

Electron-microscopic studies at first revealed only nerve fibers in the adventitia of the pial arte-

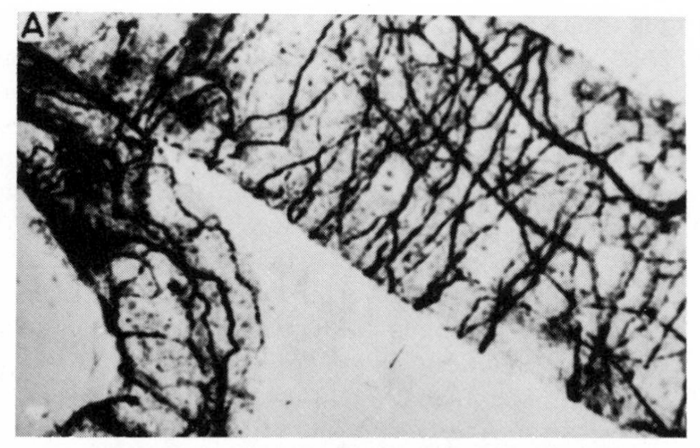

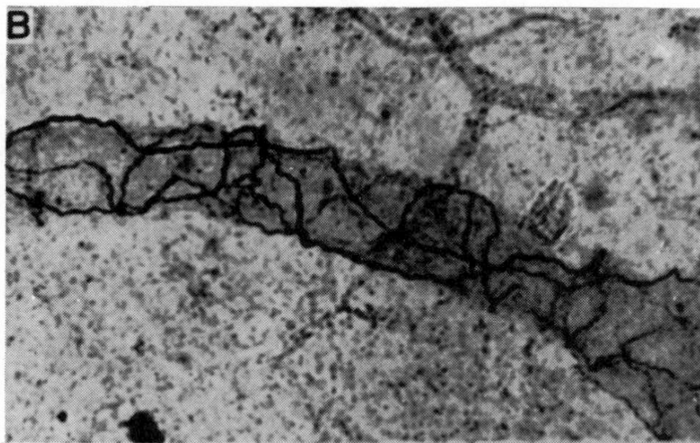

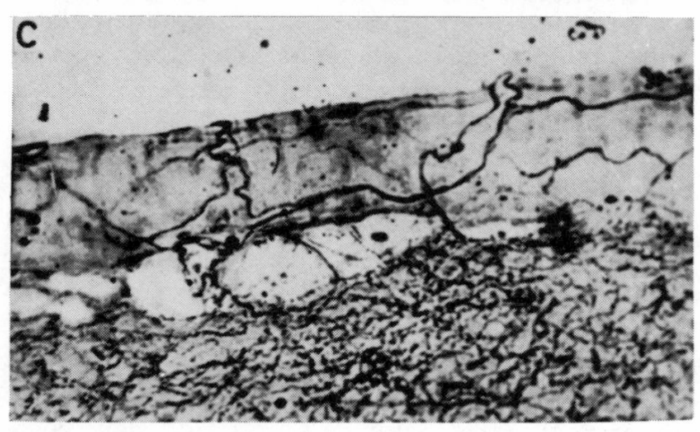

Fig. 75. Periarterial plexus of nerve fibers of pial arteries containing aceylcholinesterase. A) posterior cerebral artery of rabbit (600 μ in diameter), photomicrograph, 80X; B) branch of middle cerebral artery of rabbit (200 μ in diameter), photomicrograph, 100X; C) direct nervous connections between branch of middle cerebral artery (200 μ in diameter) and subjacent cortex in a rabbit, photomicrograph, 80X, [311].

ries, but no nerve contacts were found with the smooth-muscle cells of their walls [304]; only certain structures resembling those in the terminal membrane have been described here [49]. In a later investigation [288], both medullated and nonmedullated fibers were observed in close contact with the smooth-muscle cells; some of them evidently contained noradrenalin. More detailed investigations [131], using the electron microscope and histochemical methods, revealed nonmedullated axons with synaptic vesicles in the walls of the pial arteries in rats in the region of their contacts with smooth-muscle cells. Some of these neural structures, which disappeared after sympathectomy and administration of reserpine, are adrenergic; others are evidently cholinergic nerve fibers. Both are in close interrelationship with the smooth-muscle cells.

The writer carried out experiments on rabbits in order, first, to examine whether the dilator responses of the pial arteries caused by impulses arising from the cerebral cortex are neurogenic in origin, and second, by means of a physiological investigation, to determine the course of the nerve fibers by means of which influences from the cortex can reach the pial arteries under these conditions [249, 251]. It could be postulated that the nerve fibers conveying cortical impulses to the pial arteries are of two types: first, fibers accompanying these arteries as far as their smallest branches in the cortex, and second, fibers directly connecting the pial arteries through the pia mater with the first layer of the cortex. A microsurgical technique was developed to enable each type of nerve fiber to be divided. To exclude fibers running along the arteries, diathermy coagulation of the mouths of the radial arteries was carried under the MBS-2 stereoscopic microscope by means of a thin needle electrode at the point where they enter the brain. In another series of experiments to exclude nerve fibers connecting the pial arteries directly with the cortex, all tissue elements connecting an artery (100-120 μ in diameter) with the surrounding pia mater were carefully divided under the same microscope by means of fine glass dissecting needles. A histological control confirmed the absence of damage to the arterial walls and the underlying cortex. Responses of the pial arteries were investigated approximately 30 min or more after the operation. In these investigations, the "experimental" and "control" pial arteries were in the same cerebral hemisphere, a few milimeters apart, i.e., except for the operation, all other conditions were the same. The experiments showed that after diathermy coagulation of the mouths of radial arteries, i.e., after interruption of nerve fibers running along the vessels, postichemic (reactive) dilatation of the pial arteries developed systematically after an interruption of the cerebral circulation for 1 or 2 min. However, after division of the fibers connecting the pial

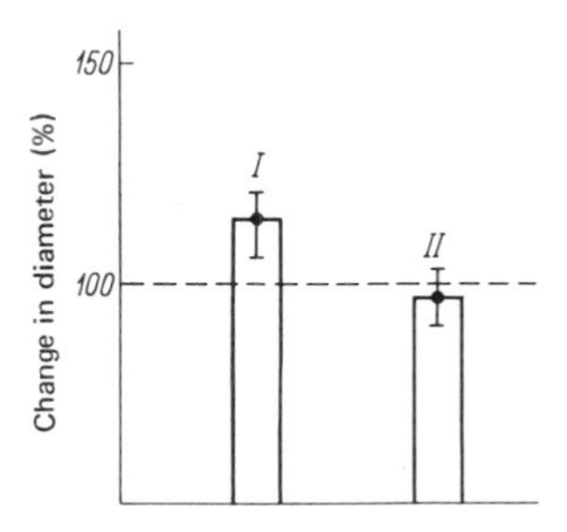

Fig. 76. Disappearance of postischemic dilatation of pial arteries of a rabbit after microsurgical division of nerve fibers connecting them directly with the cortex [249, 257]. I) Control arteries; II) "denervated" arteries. Arithmetic mean values and standard deviations shown. Initial level taken as 100%.

arteries with the surrounding pia mater, dilatation of the pial arteries did not take place, whereas adjacent (control) arteries were dilated (Fig. 76). The difference between these effects was statistically significant ($P < 0.001$). To determine whether the observed absence of responses of the pial arteries were dependent on injury to their walls during denervation, special experiments were carried out. These showed that after closure of the trachea, when carbon dioxide accumulated significantly in the arterial blood, the pial arteries dilated irrespective of whether they were intact or denervated, and the degree of dilatation was generally speaking the same. This indicates that the walls of the denervated pial arteries retain their usual reactions to hypercapnia. It can thus be concluded that in postischemic states of the brain, influences from the cortex causing dilatation of the pial arteries, when its blood supply is deficient, are apparently effected by a neurogenic mechanism. The nerve fibers responsible for this vasodilatation apparently do not run along the arteries, but through the superficial layer of the cortex and pia mater to the walls of the pial arteries.

Since the mechanisms of autoregulation may be insufficient, so that the capillary circulation in the cortex varies in response to significant changes in the systemic arterial pressure, this suggests that the responses of the pial arteries described here are, at least partially, the manifestation of a mechanism regulating an adequate inflow of blood into the cortex. For example, if the decrease in arterial pressure is not compensated in the major arteries of the brain and the blood supply to the cortex is thus reduced, the dilatation of the pial arteries which then takes place restores the cortical blood supply; the opposite chain of events takes place if the systemic arterial pressure is increased. In experiments by the author [249, 251] the dilator responses of the pial arteries to a significant decrease in the systemic arterial pressure and their vasoconstrictor responses to a corresponding increase were consistently weakened or abolished by interrupting nervous connections between the walls of blood vessels (100-200 mμ in diameter) and the cerebral cortex by means of a microsurgical operation. The results of these experiments are given in Table 8.

Further investigations of the mechanism of dilatation of the pial arteries after a stepwise decrease in the systemic arterial pressure to about 30-35 mm Hg and of the subsequent vasoconstriction following restoration of the initial level of the pressure have shown [252] that these vascular responses disappear after cerebral ischemia of 1 to 2 min duration (not because of reactive vasodilatation), to suggest a nervous rather than a muscular mechanism (i.e., caused by the Bayliss effect or by vasodilator metabolites). Intravenous administration of postganglionic cholinergic inhibitors (atropine, benactyzine, 7351) resulted in the disappear-

TABLE 8. Predominance of Active (+) or Passive (−) Response of Pial Arteries to Change in Intravascular Pressure. (Predominance of Active Response to Increased Pressure Implies: Further Constriction or Unchanged Diameter with Passive Dilatation of the Other Artery or a Lesser Degree of Passive Dilatation. The Opposite is True for Cases of Lowered Pressure).

To increase of pressure		To lowered pressure	
Intact arteries	Denervated arteries	Intact arteries	Denervated arteries
+	−	+	−
+	−	+	−
+	−	+	−
+	−	+	−
+	−	−	+
−	+	+	−
+	−	−	+
+	−	+	−
+	−	+	−
		+	−

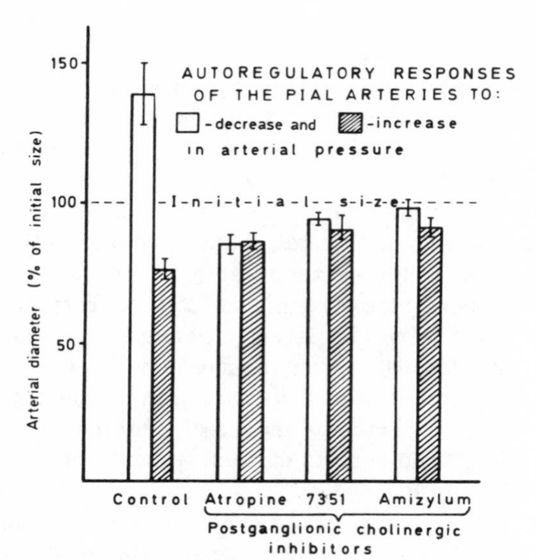

Fig. 77. Disappearance of autoregulatory dilatation of the pial arteries in response to a decrease in systemic arterial pressure from 90 ± 9.7 to 31.7 ± 7.6 mm Hg (unshaded columns) of rabbits after i.v. administration of postganglionic cholinergic inhibitors: atropine (0.2-0.3 mg/kg), 7351 (2-3 mg/kg) and benactyzine (2-3 mg/kg), while vasoconstriction after recovery of arterial pressure from 33.1 ± 7.2 to 84.6 ± 6.9 mm Hg (shaded columns) remains unchanged. Mean values and confidence limits [252].

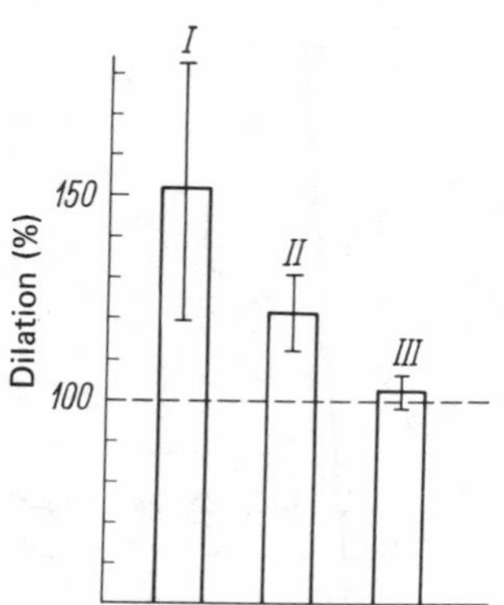

Fig. 78. Degree of dilatation of pial arteries of a rabbit during increased activity of subjacent cortex due to local application of strychnine (0.5-1.0%) [249, 251]. I) When cortical blood supply is deficient following coagulation of mouths of radial arteries, effect is increased; II) control arteries; III) after microsurgical division of nerve fibers connecting pial arteries with cortex, as a rule vasodilatation is absent. Arithmetic mean values and standard deviations given. Original diameter taken as 100%.

ance of autoregulatory vasodilatation while vasoconstriction remained unchanged (Fig. 77). Similar results were obtained when benactyzine and 7351 were applied locally to the brain surface. Experimental analysis proved the specificity of the effects of the drugs mentioned. The conclusion is that a nervous cholinergic mechanism is involved in the functional dilatation of the pial arteries in response to a decreased blood supply to the cerebral cortex.

Evidence has also been obtained which indicates that nervous mechanisms may participate in the genesis of functional vasodilatation in the brain following an increase in cortical electrical activity. The fact that the dilatation of the pial arteries occurs before an increase of electrical activity suggests that dilatation of the pial arteries is not due to the action of cortical metabolites on the vessel walls, but that its mechanism is more likely to be neurogenic. On the other hand, interruption of nervous connections between the cortex and pial arteries by the above-mentioned technique abolished vasodilatation in response to increased cortical activity [249, 251]. The experiments showed that after diathermy coagulation of the mouths of the radial arteries, i.e., after interruption of nerve fibers running along the vessels, the dilator responses of the pial arteries to application of strychnine and the corresponding changes in the electrocorticogram did not disappear, but on the contrary, they frequently were increased. In these experiments the control arteries were dilated by 21 ± 9%, and the denervated arteries by 51 ± 32% ($M \pm \sigma$); the apparent explanation of this fact is that because of occlusion of the radial arteries an additional deficiency of blood supply to the cortex was produced, leading to dilatation of the pial arteries. However, after interruption of the nervous connections between the pial arteries (with a caliber of 100-200 μ) and the surrounding pia mater, their dilator response usually disappeared or was so weak as to be negligible (Fig. 78). Consequently, when the activity of the cortex was increased, just as when its blood supply was insufficient, the dilator responses of the pial arteries disappeared after separation of their walls from the surrounding pial tissues. As was pointed out above, this absence of response of the pial arteries was not connected with injury to their walls during denervation.

The dilatation of the pial arteries that regularly followed asphyxia or microsurgical division of nerve fibers connecting the pial arteries to the first layer of the cortex was not abolished, and the degree of dilatation of intact and, "denervated" arteries was generally speaking the same (18 and 20% on the average respectively; difference not statistically significant, $P > 0.5$); however, it was observed that dilatation of the denervated arteries usually occurred later than that of the adjacent control vessels [249, 251]. These findings indicated that the action of CO_2 on the arterial walls from inside the lumen may be direct, but under normal conditions a definite role in the production of vasodilatation is played by nerve impulses reaching the pial arteries from the cortex. As has been shown above, the action of CO_2 on the cerebral vessels may be not only direct, but also indirect, through the intervention of vasomotor nervous influences.

In experiments on rabbits, after intravenous injection of atropine, which blocks muscarine-like cholinergic receptors in blood vessel walls [13], in a dose of 0.1 mg/kg body weight the dilator response of the pial arteries to direct application of strychnine to the cerebral cortex was weakened: whereas the arteries in the control dilated by $31 \pm 2.6\%$ of their initial diameter, after treatment with atropine the vasodilatation was only $11 \pm 2\%$ ($P < 0.001$). The same results in general were obtained by the use of other muscarine-like cholinolytic drugs (methyldiazine, fubromegan, 7351, etc.). These findings indicate that both adrenergic and cholinergic mechanisms may have a role in the mechanism of functional dilatation of the pial arteries, although further investigation of this problem is necessary.

There is thus considerable experimental evidence at the present time to indicate that the mechanism of functional vasodilatation of the pial arteries is neurogenic: 1) the vascular response precedes the increase in cortical electrical activity and diminishes when electrical activity is at its highest level; this is evidence against the view that vasodilation is entirely the result of the action of metabolites on the vessel walls; 2) microsurgical interruption of nerve fibers connecting the pial arteries with the cortex abolishes their dilator response; 3) adrenergic and cholinergic structures can be demonstrated histochemically in the walls of the pial arteries; some cholinolytic drugs reduce the functional dilatation of the pial arteries, suggesting that neural mechanism participates in the vascular response. However, many aspects of this problem of the physiological mechanisms of functional vasodilatation in the brain unexplained and require further experimental investigation. The possibility is not ruled out that further research will reveal a definite role of both nervous and humoral mechanisms in its production, supplementing or replacing each other under certain conditions.

The possibility of a nervous mechanism of the responses of the pial arteries may appear to contradict the well-established fact that the arteries react only weakly to direct action of adrenalin, noradrenalin, and acetylcholine, which play an important role in the transmission of nerve impulses to the smooth muscle cells of the vascular media. After local application of adrenalin to the brain surface, of cats slight constriction (not more than 3-30% of their initial size) of the pial arteries more than 50 μ in diameter was observed [80, 76]. In the present author's experiments the direct effect of adrenalin and noradrenalin on the pial arteries was also inconstant and slight. In response to the direct action of acetylcholine on the pial arteries the effect was weak and inconstant [364]. The writer's previous experiments also showed that the pial arteries of rabbits respond to the direct action of acetylcholine in some cases by dilatation, in others by constriction, while in a third group of cases they do not respond at all. It could be supposed that in response to direct application of acetylcholine and other physiologically active substances to the brain surface, the response of the pial arteries, which seem to be the main factor regulating the inflow of blood into the cortex, is largely determined by the metabolic needs of the cortical tissues and, consequently, by the character of the cortical effects on the pial arteries. Later investigations carried out on rabbits [249, 251] to test the direct action of acetylcholine (in dilutions of 1×10^{-4}-1×10^{-6}) in fact showed that under ordinary conditions dilatation of intact pial arteries measuring 100-200 μ in diameter was slight (on the average by $8 \pm 4\%$). After microcoagulation of the mouths of all radial arteries (when the cortex begin to experience a deficiency of its blood supply) the dilator response of these same pial arteries to acetylcholine was increased sharply (dilatation by $58 \pm 6.8\%$). When, on the other hand, nerve fibers connecting the pial arteries to the cortex were interrupted microsurgically (see above), dilatation of these arteries from application of acetylcholine again was slight (by $11 \pm 6.5\%$) (Fig. 79). The results of these experiments, first, explain to some extent the reason for the weak and inconstant reaction of the pial arteries to the direct action of physiologically active substances:

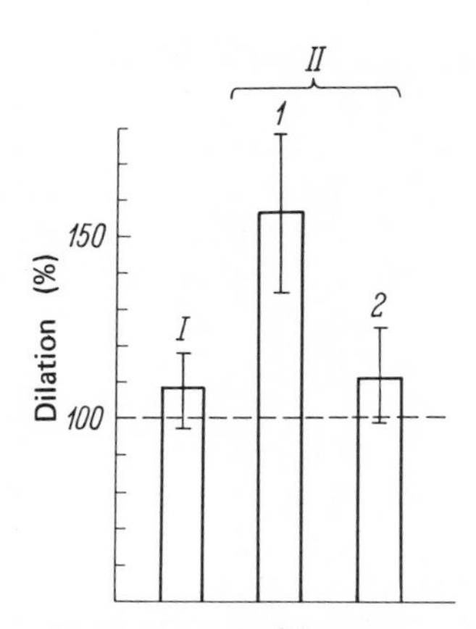

Fig. 79. Increase in dilator response of pial arteries of a rabbit to direct action of acetylcholine in the presence of an inadequate cortical blood supply, and disappearance of this increase after microsurgical division of nerve connections between pial arteries and cortex [249, 251]. I) Normal conditions; II) deficient cortical blood supply after coagulation of mouths of all radial arteries: 1) pial arteries with intact nerve connections with cortex, 2) pial arteries after division of these connections. Arithmetic mean values and standard deviations shown. Original level taken as 100%. Details given in text.

the reactivity of the walls of these vessels is determined by the metabolic needs of that part of the cortex which they supply with blood. Second, these experiments show that cortical influences determining the reactivity of the pial arteries to the action of physiologically active substances are effected by nerve fibers running from the cortex to the pial arteries lying on its surface.

An attempt was also made to examine the physiological mechanism of dilatation of the pial arteries which brings about the collateral inflow of blood into the bed of the occluded vessel. First, this dilatation peripherally to the site of occlusion could be a myogenic reaction of the arterial wall in response to a fall of intravascular pressure, i.e., a Bayliss effect, as has been postulated in the case of reactive (postischemic) hyperemia in other organs [15, 78]; second, the dilator response of the pial arteries could be due to the accumulation of carbon dioxide in the brain tissues; third, dilatation of the pial arteries could be neurogenic in origin. This problem was investigated experimentally [239, 240], with the following results:

1. Repeated (after 4-7 min) cauterization of the wall of a pial artery with the needle of a galvanocautery immediately peripherally to the site of occlusion (when no changes could have occurred in the intravascular pressure or an excess of CO_2 could have accumulated in the brain tissue), caused dilatation of the artery and of its branches (Fig. 80A). This indicated that the dilator response of the pial arteries described above is neither the result of accumulation of CO_2 in the region of the vessel wall, nor a myogenic Bayliss effect, but that it must evidently be neurogenic. The results of this experiment also did not support the view that dilatation of the arteries is neuroparalytic, i.e., is dependent on injury to the nerve fibers running along the pial arteries from the larger to the smaller branches.

2. If the conduction of nerve impulses along the nerve fibers running along the wall of an artery is blocked by the strictly local application of 20% formalin solution in alcohol over a distance of 300-500 μ (which leaves the blood flow in the vessel undisturbed), and occlusion of the artery is produced proximally, the branches of the arteries lying distally to the point of application are not dilated; however, after repeated occlusion of the same artery peripherally to the zone treated with formalin, a typical dilator response of all its branches develops (Fig. 80B). This is also evidence of a neurogenic mechanism of the dilator response of the artery.

3. After cauterization of the pia close to an artery with the needle electrode of a diathermy cautery (at a distance of 30-50 μ from the vessel wall, when the wall of the artery was undamaged and the blood flow in it remained intact), a typical dilator response of all branches of this artery located peripherally relative to the blood flow was observed (Fig. 80C). This could be neither a Bayliss effect nor the result of accumulation of CO_2 in the brain tissue, but it was most probably a neurogenic dilator response of the pial arteries to stimulation of nervous structures in the pia connected with vascular nerves.

The results of all these experiments show that active dilatation of the pial arteries peripherally to the site of occlusion (dilatation of the whole system of branches and activation of hitherto not functioning anastomoses) is due neither to a Bayliss effect nor to diffusion of metabolites from the ischemic brain tissue in the region of the arterial walls (or at least, not only to these mechanisms), but develops by a neurogenic mechanism. In cases of coagulation of the pial arteries by galvanic or diathermy currents, impulses spread from the region of occlusion to the small arterial branches and anastomoses located peripherally.

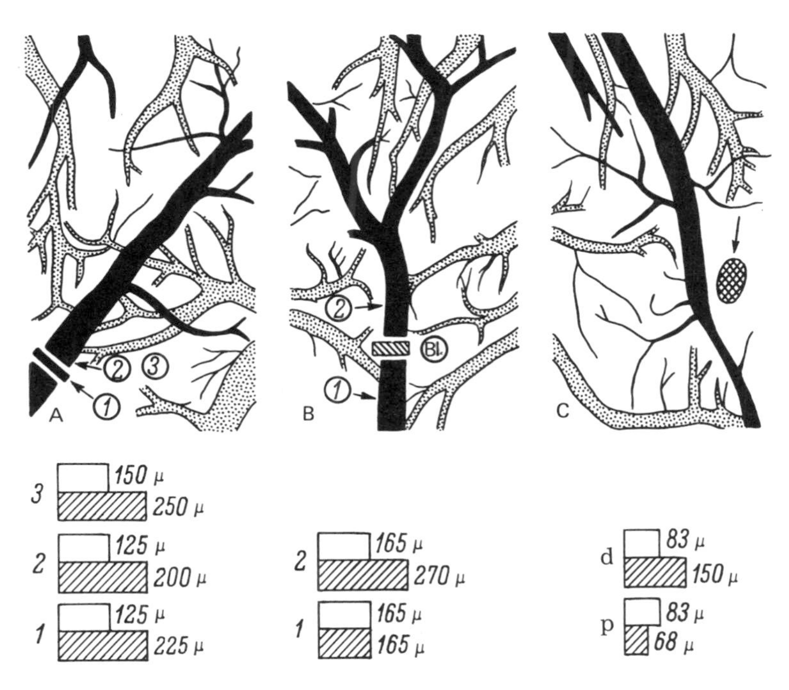

Fig. 80. Scheme of experiments indicating a neurogenic mechanism of dilatation of the pial arteries peripherally to the site of occlusion [240]. Columns below the diagrams of the pial vessels denote diameters of arteries in microns before (unshaded) and after (shaded) procedure. A) After repeated cauterizations of the arterial wall peripherally to the site of occlusion (1) at intervals of 5-10 min (2 and 3) it again dilates. B) After occlusion of the artery before the site of the blocking of conduction of impulses along the arterial wall (Bl.) dilator response of peripheral segments is absent (1); when the artery was occluded peripherally to the site of the block (Bl.), dilatation is present (2). C) After cauterization of the pia close to the artery (indicated by an arrow), a typical dilator response of the distal (d) segment of the artery developed (above), while its proximal (p) segment (below). on the other hand, became constricted. Explanation in text.

The results of experiments by other researchers [379] also suggested that metabolites diffusing from the tissues should play no part in the development of this vascular response. First, the latent period of the collateral inflow of blood, measured by thermistors (1-4 sec) is much shorter than the time taken for appreciable changes to develop in the CO_2 tension and pH in the brain tissues. This difference could not be due to inertia of the selective electrodes used, and it is on the whole doubtful that metabolites could accumulate in such a short time. Second, the accumulation of CO_2 and change in pH must be maximal in the focus of ischemia and must diminish progressively from it toward the periphery. These workers also doubt that metabolites could spread so rapidly into the region of blood vessels which are not yet affected by ischemic changes but which participate in the collateral circulation. The possibility of CO_2 accumulation and the Bayliss effect in zones of mixed circulation was denied also in earlier papers [264]. However, although rejecting any possible role of metabolites or of the Bayliss effect, Meyer and co-workers [379] nevertheless did not then accept that the mechanism of vasodilatation of the cerebral vessels responsible for the collateral circulation could be neurogenic in character. Nevertheless, in the discussion at the Symposium on Correlation of Blood Supply with Metabolism and Function (Tbilisi, 1968) on the problem of nervous control of the cerebral circulation (after the paper by Moskalenko et al. [280]) Meyer concluded that there is now substantial evidence for this view: "1. No other explanation is as satisfactory. The opposite view, that they are secondary to metabolic changes from EEG activation, is unsatisfactory since regional increases in cerebral blood flow dependent on metabolic factors take several seconds to become evident. 2. These rhythmic fluctuations in pO_2 of the gray matter are diffuse throughout the brain in the steady state suggesting some central controlling influences. 3. They are abolished by CO_2 inhalation and anything that destroys autoregulation or vasomotor reactivity. 4. Evidence (to be discussed later in this symposium) regarding sleep indicates that exceedingly rapid, brief, and large changes in cerebral blood flow occur during rapid eye movement (REM) sleep. 5. The innervation of the cerebral vessels would be adequate to account for vasomotor control by the cerebral cortex. 6. Stimulation of the reticular formation in the brain stem sometimes causes EEG changes and an increase in cerebral blood flow without an increase in cerebral oxygen consumption, although the latter usually occurred'' ([280], pp. 163-164).

Thus, although the idea of a nervous mechanism controlling the functional behavior of small cerebral arteries was previously completely rejected by the majority of researchers, the experimental evidence now increasingly indicates that such a mechanism must play an important role in the regulation of an adequate blood supply to the brain tissue.

CONCLUDING REMARKS

The function of the circulatory system in the widest sense is to provide adequate microcirculation in every part of the body. The intensity of the capillary circulation in any part of the brain, for instance, is determined by the overall pressure gradient in its vascular system and also by the total resistance from the aorta to that particular capillary network (the capillaries and veins play a minor role in the regulation of cerebrovascular resistance. Investigation of functional behavior of different parts of the vascular system and its effect on the cerebral hemodynamics is nothing more than the study of the microcirculation in the brain in the broad meaning of this concept [302]. In this book an attempt has been made to generalize the results of research of this type into the cerebral circulation. It includes an account of all that has so far been discovered concerning the functional behavior of different parts of the cerebrovascular system during regulation or pathological changes of the cerebral circulation. This type of investigation of the cerebral circulation is as yet only in its infancy, and the reader who has taken note of the experimental data described in this book will be able to assess for himself how far it was possible to resolve the problems concerned with normal and pathological physiology at the present state of study of this subject.

In the first half of this century, many experimental facts were discovered which demonstrated the active role of the vascular system of the brain in the regulation of its circulation. However, in cases when the methods used yielded quantitative data (and unfortunately, in most cases this was impossible), it was found that all nervous effects and most humoral effects on the cerebral vessels were extremely weak. If these effects were always as weak as this, regulation of the cerebral circulation would be impossible. On the other hand, the absence of lucid results of these experimental investigations itself provided sufficient grounds for the conclusion that nervous control over the cerebral circulation is in fact absent or nearly so; however, it could equally indicate that the methods used for its detection were unsuitable for the purpose. For example, it could be claimed that the artificial stimulation or division of the vascular nerves, as usually used to investigate these problems, like the direct application of neurohumoral agents to the vessels (externally or internally), could only disturb the normal circulation in the brain. Quite logically it was suggested that under these conditions the mechanisms of regulation of the circulation in the brain which have developed in the course of evolution are more refined than those in other parts of the body, and they quickly correct experimentally induced disturbances of the normal circulation; for this reason experimental results have so far proved unclear or even negative. Accordingly, at the first stage of his investigations of the cerebral circulation the present author reached the following conclusion: that in order to explain more easily how the vessels regulating the circulation work, and how their functional behavior differs, it was essential to carry out the investigations under conditions when the mechanisms of regulation of the cerebral circulation are functioning naturally, i.e., are either adapting the circulation of blood in the brain to changes in the metabolic cemands of its tissues or are compensating disturbances of the cerebral circulation. To this end, in some experiments various disorders of the circulation of blood in the brain were produced and under these circumstances, the behavior of different parts of the cerebrovascular system, including the major arterial trunks and the pial and intracerebral arteries, was studied and the changes taking place in the cerebral circulation were observed. It seemed to the present author that his investigations would most conveniently be started with pathological conditions, because this would provide a particularly wide range of conditions under which the operation of mechanisms controlling the circulation in the brain could be detected. When, on the other hand, the general character of behavior of the different cerebral vessels had been discovered, in order to analyze the phenomena physiological methods such as stimulation and division of vascular nerves, the direct action of neurohumoral agents on the vessels, and so on, could be used in addition. This, in broad outline, was the plan followed by the author in his investigations of the cerebral circulation.

Since few systematic studies have so far been carried out in this direction, the problems largely remain unsolved. Nevertheless, the available experimental data have already shed considerable light on the character of functional behavior of different parts of the cerebrovascular system; they have clearly demonstrated that the role of the vessels of the brain in regulation of the cerebral circulation in many cases requires the participation of neurogenic mechanisms (although the participation of purely humoral mechanisms likewise cannot yet be ruled out). However, these vasomotor mechanisms in the brain have so far received very little study, so that in most cases neither their receptive zones, nor their nervous pathways, nor the localization of the central coordinating systems of these reflexes are known.

At the present stage of research into the cerebral circulation, it has been possible to obtain new facts only through the use of many different methods giving direct and, where possible, quantitative information on the functional behavior of individual parts of the vascular system and on the hemodynamics in the brain. This was absolutely essential because the principal controllable function in the cerebral circulatory system, i.e., the capillary circulation of the brain, is dependent on many variables. In order to analyze this function, experimental conditions had to be created under which as many influences as possible could be considered together; in addition, it was sometimes necessary to stabilize some parameters in order to study changes in others. All these considerations frequently called for highly complex experimental conditions and, in particular, for several types of operations. The possibility cannot be ignored that this, in turn, could be reflected in the animal's general condition and, consequently, that it could modify the normal functional behavior of the vascular mechanisms of the brain. The least of the evils had to be chosen: each experiment had to be so designed that it would give the fullest possible information on the observed phenomenon, but at the same time, attempts were made to ensure that the functional behavior of the vascular mechanisms of the brain would be undisturbed. It was also necessary to insist that hypotheses found their correct place in the research – that they remained inside the laboratory where they could assist in the correct organization of experiments, and where there was no risk of their replacing the results of experimental research.

During his investigations into the regulation and disorders of the cerebral circulation, the author has endeavored to publish their results only when they would shed fresh light on the respective problems and provide new facts to assist the explanation of the processes taking place in the cerebral circulatory system. In his generalization of the experimental material on each aspect of the problem the author has always striven to avoid complex logical constructions in which theoretical conclusions are widely divorced from the experimental data. On the one hand, the experiments were planned as far as possible in order to give straight answers to specific problems. On the other hand, the author has endeavored only to draw conclusions which emerge directly from the experimental findings. This may perhaps to some extent explain why, despite the evident novelty of most of the conclusions, the results of subsequent investigations in his own laboratory, as well as the findings obtained by other workers published in the scientific press, as a rule have only confirmed the earlier conclusions.

In his studies of the cerebral circulation the author has always endeavored to arrange the problems for study in their correct order and not to anticipate, not to tackle one problem until the one before it is solved. This is, of course, a general principle of development of every branch of science, but it is the *conditio sine qua non* when any individual problem, including the cerebral circulation, is studied. For example, nervous control over the cerebral circulation and correlation between blood supply and function of the brain could be considered only after a solution had been found to the problem of the functional behavior of those vessels on which vasomotor nervous impulses can act, or which participate in the regulation of an adequate blood supply to the brain.

One aspect of the problem of the cerebral circulation which still remains, and one which is of considerable importance, is that of peculiarities in its mechanism of regulation in different parts of the brain. The brain, of course, consists essentially of a large number of "organs," whose functions, and their related metabolism and blood supply, may vary relatively independently. This can take place under physiological conditions, but it does so to a far greater degree in disease. It is well known that the anatomical structure of the vascular system varies in different parts of the brain; nevertheless, the characteristics of the physiology and regulation of the circulation, as they vary in different parts of the central nervous system, still await study. It is clear that much time and much combined effort on the part of neurophysiologists, neurobiochemists, neuromorphologists, and specialists in circulatory studies will be required before these problems are finally solved.

BIBLIOGRAPHY

1. Ageichenko, F. E., "On nerve cells in the leptomeninges," Arkh. Patol., 18(1):21 (1956).
2. Aleksandrovskaya, M. M., Vascular Changes in the Brain in Various Pathological States, Moscow (1965).
3. Amashukeli, G. V., "Analysis of circulatory changes in the brain in hemorrhage and hemotransfusion," Patol. Fiziol. i Éxper. Terap., 13(3):29 (1969).
4. Ames, A., Wright, L., Kowada, M., Thurston, J., and Majno, G., "Cerebral ischemia. II. The no-reflow phenomenon," Amer. J. Pathol., 52:437 (1968).
5. Antoshkina, E. D., and Naumenko, A. I., "Changes in blood supply of the cortical ends of the visual and auditory analyzers during stimulation," Fiziol. Zh. SSSR, 46:1305 (1960).
6. Ask-Upmark, E., The Carotid Sinus and the Cerebral Circulation, Copenhagen (1935).
7. Austin, G. M., Corson, R., Linder, J., Chamberlain, R., and Grant, F. C., "Cerebral edema: studies on its location and mode of action with radioactive sodium," Arch. Neurol. Psychiat. (Chicago), 75:447 (1956).
8. Ayala, G. F., and Himwich, W. A., "Middle cerebral and lingual artery pressure in the dog," Arch. Neurol. (Chicago), 12:435 (1965).
9. Bakay, L., "Studies on the blood-brain barrier with radioactive phosphorus. V. Effect of cerebral injuries and infection on the barrier," Arch. Neurol. Psychiat. (Chicago), 73:2 (1955).
10. Bakay, L., and Lee, J., Cerebral Edema, Thomas, Springfield (Illinois) (1965).
11. Baramidze, D. G., "A technique for studying the structure and functional states of cerebral blood vessels," Soobshch. Akad. Nauk Gruz. SSR, 44:491 (1966).
12. Baramidze, D. G., and Mchedlishvili, G. I., "Arrangement and responses of smooth muscle cells in the arterial walls of the cerebral cortex," Byull. Éxperim. Biol. i Med., 68(11):112 (1970).
13. Barlow, R., Introduction to Chemical Pharmacology, Methuen, London (1955).
14. Baron, M. A., "Cerebral meninges. Histology and physiology," in: Great Medical Encyclopedia, Second Edition, 18:847 Moscow (1960).
15. Bayliss, W. M., "On the local reactions of the arterial wall to changes of internal pressure," J. Physiol. (London), 28:220 (1902).
16. Benua, N. N., "On the regional cerebral blood flow in the visual cortex," in: Kedrov, A. A. (ed.), Problems of the Physiology of the Cerebral Circulation, Leningrad (1970), pp. 34-52.
17. Beranek, R., Fantiš, A., Gutmann, E., and Vrbova, H., "Postoperative edema of the brain," Czech. Fiziol., 1(2):142 (1952).
18. Beranek, R., Fantiš, A., Gutmann, E., and Vrbova, G., Pokusné Studie o Mozkovém Edemu, Praha (1955).
19. Betz, E., "pH-abhängige Regulationen der lokalen Gehirndurchblutung," in: Hydrodynamik, Elektrolyt- und Saure-Basen-Haushalt im Liquor und Nervensystem, Stuttgart (1967), pp. 17-27.
20. Betz. E., und Kozak, R., "Der Einfluss der Wasserstoffionenkonzentration der Gehirnrinde auf die Regulation der corticalen Durchblutung," Pflügers Arch. ges. Physiol., 293:56 (1967).
21. Betz, E., Kozak, R., and Heredia, A., "Die Bedeutung der pH der Gehirnrinder für die Regulation der kortikalen Durchblutung." Pflügers Arch. ges. Physiol. 289:23 (1966).
22. Biedl, A., and Reiner, M., "Studien über Hirncirculation und Hirnödem," Pflügers Arch. ges. Physiol., 79:158 (1900).
23. Biryukov, D. A., "Depressor reflex of the blood pressure in response to mechanical stimulation of the dura," Fiziol. Zh. SSSR, 34:689 (1948).
24. Blinova, A. M., and Ryzhova, N. M., "Blood supply of the brain during reflex action. Report 3. Role of the carotid sinus zones in reg-

ulation of the blood supply of the brain during stimulation of interoceptors," Byull. Éksperim. Biol. i Med., 44(12):3 (1957).

25. Blinova, A. M., and Ryzhova, N. M., "The role of anastomoses between branches of the external and internal carotid arteries for the blood supply to the brain," Byull. Éksperim. Biol. i Med., 52(8):3 (1961).

26. Blinova, A. M., and Ryzhova, N. M., "Nervous regulation of the blood supply to the brain," Vestn. Akad. Med. Nauk SSSR, No. 5, p. 56 (1961).

27. Bloch, E. H., "Microscopic observations of the circulating blood in the bulbar conjunctiva in man in health and disease," Ergebn. Anat. Entw.-Gesch., 36:1 (1956).

28. Bogomolez, A., "Über den Blutbruck in den kleinen Arterien und Venen (den Kapillaren nahestehenden) unter normalen und gewissen pathologischen Verhältnissen," Pflügers Arch. ges. Physiol., 141:118 (1911).

29. Bol'shakov, O. P., "On the significance of pulsating volume changes in the internal carotid artery for venous blood flow in the dural sinuses," in: Konradi, G. P. (ed.), Mechanisms of the Neurohumoral Control of Vegetative Functions, Leningrad (1970), pp. 12-17.

30. Borodula, A. V., "Morphology of the nervous apparatus of the normal human internal carotid artery," Zh. Nevropat. i Psikhiat., 65:379 (1965).

31. Borodula, A. V., "Morphology of the nervous apparatus of the internal carotid artery," in: Vascular Diseases of the Brain, No. 2. Proceedings of the 4th All-Union Congress of Neuropathologists and Psychiatrists, Vol. 2, Moscow (1965), pp. 336-343.

32. Bouckaert, J. J., and Heymans, C., "Carotid sinus reflexes, influence of central blood pressure and blood supply on respiratory and vasomotor centers," J. Physiol. (London), 79:49 (1933).

33. Bouckaert, J. J., and Heymans, C., "On the reflex regulation of the cerebral blood flow and the cerebral vasomotor tone," J. Physiol. (London), 84:367 (1935).

34. Bozzao, L., Fieschi, C., Agnoli, A., and Nardini, M., "Autoregulation of cerebral blood flow studied in the brain of cat," in: Bain, H., and Harper, A. M. (eds.), Blood Flow through Organs and Tissues, Edinburgh and London (1968), pp. 253-257.

35. Braasch, D., and Henning, W., "Erythrocytenflexibilität und Strömungswiderstand in Capillaren mit einem Durchmesser unter 20 μ," Pflügers Arch. ges. Physiol., 286:76 (1965).

36. Braasch, D., "Erythrocyte flexibility and blood flow resistance in capillaries with a diameter of less than 20 microns," in: Harders, H. (ed.), 4th European Conference on Microcirculation, Karger, Phiebig, Basel–New York (1967), pp. 272-275.

37. Brain, S. R., "Order and disorder in the cerebral circulation," Lancet, No. 7001, p. 857 (1957).

38. Broman, T., Über cerebrale Zirkulationsstörungen, Copenhagen (1940).

39. Byrom, F. B., "The pathogenesis of hypertensive encephalopathy and its relation to the malignant phase of hypertension," Lancet, No. 6831, p. 201 (1954).

40. Carlyle, A., and Grayson, J., "Factors involved in the control of the cerebral blood flow," J. Physiol. (London), 133:10 (1956).

41. Carpi, A., and Virno, M., "Interaction between the electrical activity and the circulation of the brain: significance of metabolic and humoral factors under various conditions of functional activity," in: Meyer, J. S., and Gastaut, H. (eds.), Cerebral Anoxia and the Electroencephalogram, Thomas, Springfield (1961), pp. 112-117.

42. Chiang, J., Kowada, M., Ames, A., Wright, L., and Majno, G., "Cerebral ischemia. III. Vascular changes," Amer. J. Pathol., 52:455 (1968).

43. Chorobski, J., and Penfield, W., "Cerebral vasodilator nerves and their pathway from the medulla oblongata," Arch. Neurol. Psychiat. (Chicago), 28:1257 (1932).

44. Clark, M. E., Martin, J. D., Wenglarz, R. A., Himwich, W. A., and Knapp, F. M., "Engineering analysis of the hemodynamics of the circle of Willis," Arch. Neurol. (Chicago) 13:173 (1965).

45. Cooper, R., Crow, H. J., Walter, W. G., and Winter, A. L., "Regional control of cerebral reactivity and oxygen supply in brain," Brain Res., 3:174 (1966).

46. Corday, E., Rothenberg, S. F., and Putnam, T. J., "Cerebral vascular insufficiency. An explanation of some types of localized cerebral encephalopathy," Arch. Neurol. Psychiat. (Chicago), 69:551 (1953).

47. Corday, E., Rothenberg, S. F., and Weiner, S. M., "Cerebral vascular insufficiency. An explanation of the transient stroke," Arch. Intern. Med.. 98:683 (1956).

48. Cushing, H., "Some experimental and clinical observations concerning states of increased intracranial pressure," Amer. J. Med. Sci., 124:375 (1902).
49. Dahl, E., and Nelson, E. "Electron microscopic observation on human intracranial arteries. II. Innervation," Arch. Neurol. (Chicago), 10:158 (1964).
50. Davydov, I. N., "Further investigations into the dynamics of the cerebral circulation during exposure to factors of the internal milieu of the body. Proceedings of the 22nd Scientific Session," Tr. Volgogradsk. Gos. Med. Inst., 16:144 (1964).
51. Decker, E., and Hipp, E., "Der vasale Gefässkranz. Morphologie und Angiologie," Anat. Anz., 105(6-9):100 (1958).
52. Dickinson, C. J., Neurogenic Hypertension, Davis, Philadelphia (1965).
53. Dieckhoff, D., and Kanzow, E., "Über die Lokalisation des Strömungswiderstandes im Hirnkreislauf," Pflügers Arch. ges. Physiol., 310:75 (1969).
54. Dmitrieva, T. D., "Effect of proprioception on some indices of the cerebral circulation," in: Pathogenesis, Clinical Features, Treatment, and Prophylaxis of the Most Important Diseases, Volgograd (1963), pp. 117-119.
55. Dobrovol'tseva-Zaitseva, E. A., "Innervation of arteries of the human brain," Arkh. Anat., Gistol., i Émbriol., 26(6):72 (1950).
56. Donders, F. C., "Die Bewegungen des Gehirns und die Veränderungen der Gefässfüllung der Pia Mater," Schmid's Jahrbücher, 69:16 (1851).
57. Dotsenko, A. P., "Changes in the permeability of the blood-brain barrier in closed head injuries," Dokl. Akad. Nauk SSSR, 120:673 (1958).
58. Dozio, C., Fumicalli, B., and Noll, S., "Preparato cuore-pulmoni-testa isolati di mammifero per la studio del circolo cerebrale," Boll. Soc. Ital. Biol. Sper., 33:1036 (1957).
59. Dukes, H. T., and Viet, R. G., "Cerebral arteriography during migraine prodrome and headache," Neurology 14:636 (1964).
60. Dzhavakhishvili, N. A., "Development of the vessels of the human brain in the second half of intrauterine life," Transactions of the Institute of Experimental Morphology, Academy of Sciences of the Georgian SSR, Vol. 5., Tbilisi (1965), pp. 26-35.
61. Echlin, F. A., "Vasospasm and focal cerebral ischemia," Arch. Neurol. Psychiat. (Chicago), 47:77 (1942).
62. Egorov, B. G., and Kandel', É. I., "Prophylaxis and treatment of edema and swelling of the brain and acute circulatory disturbances after brain injury," Vopr. Neirokhir., No. 2, p. 3 (1958).
63. Ekström-Jodal, B., Häggendal, E., Nilsson, N. J., and Norbäck, B., "Changes of the transmural pressure – the probable stimulus to cerebral blood flow autoregulation," in: Brock, M. et al. (eds.), Cerebral Blood Flow, Berlin–Heidelberg–New York (1969), pp. 89-93.
64. Erkhov, I. S., "The problem of innervation of the intracerebral vessels," in: Acute Disturbances of the Cerebral Circulation, Moscow (1960), pp. 531-538.
65. Erkhov, I. S., "Material on innervation of the intracerebral vessels," in: Vascular Diseases of the Brain, No. 2, Proceedings of the 4th All-Union Congress of Neuropathologists and Psychiatrists, Vol. 2, Moscow (1965), pp. 333-336.
66. Fahraeus, R., and Lindqvist, T., "The viscosity of the blood in narrow capillary tubes," Amer. J. Physiol., 96:562 (1931).
67. Falck, B., Mchedlishvili, G. I., and Owman, C., "Histochemical demonstration of adrenergic nerves in cortex-pia of rabbit," Acta Pharmacol., 23:133 (1965).
68. Fang, H. C. H., "Cerebral arterial innervation in man," Arch. Neurol., 4:651 (1961).
69. Field, E. J., Grayson, J., and Rogers, A. F., "Observations on the blood flow in the spinal cord of the rabbit," J. Physiol. (London), 114:56 (1951).
70. Fields, W. S., Elwards, W. H., and Crawford, E. S., "Bilateral carotid artery thrombosis," Arch. Neurol. (Chicago), 4:369 (1961).
71. Filatov, A. I., Pashkovsky, E. V., and Tsybulyak, G. N., "Cerebral microcirculation changes in acute blood losses and prolonged hypotension," Byull. Éxperim. Biol. i. Med., 69(1):20 (1970).
72. Finnerty, F. A., Witkin, L., and Fazekas, J. F., "Cerebral hemodynamics during cerebral ischemia induced by acute hypotension," J. Clin. Invest., 33:1227 (1954).
73. Fischer, H., "Verlauf und Form der Hirnarterien und ihre funktionelle Bedeutung," I. Mitteilung. Verh. Anat. Ges. Supplement to Vol. 100, Jena (1954), pp. 355-361.
74. Florey, H., "Microscopical observations on the circulation of the blood in the cerebral cortex," Brain, 48:43 (1925).
75. Fog, M., "Cerebral circulation. The reaction of the pial arteries to a fall of blood pressure," Arch. Neurol. Psychiat. (Chicago), 37:351 (1937).

76. Fog. M., "Cerebral circulation, II. Reaction of pial arteries to increase in blood pressure." Arch. Neurol. Psychiat. (Chicago) 41:260 (1939)
77. Fog, M., "Autoregulation of cerebral blood flow and its abolition by local hypoxia and/or trauma," in: International Symposium on CBF and CSF. Scand. J. Lab. and Clin. Invest., Suppl. 102, V-B (1968).
78. Folkow, B., "Intravascular pressure as a factor regulating the tone of the small vessels," Acta Physiol. Scand., 17:289 (1949).
79. Forbes, H. S., Mason, G. I., and Wortman, R. C., "Cerebral circulation. XLIV. Vasodilatation in the pia following stimulation of the vagus, aortic, and carotid sinus nerves," Arch. Neurol. Psychiat. (Chicago), 37:334 (1937).
80. Forbes, H. S., and Wolff, H. G., "Cerebral circulation. III. The vasomotor control of cerebral vessels," Arch. Neurol. Psychiat. (Chicago), 19:1057 (1928).
81 Fraser, R. A. R., Stein, B. M., Barret, R. E., and Pool, J. L., "Noradrenergic mediation of experimental cerebrovascular spasm," Stroke, 1:356 (1970).
82. Freeman, J., "Elimination of brain cortical blood flow autoregulation following hypoxia," in: International Symposium on CBF and CSF. Scand. J. Lab. Clin. Invest., Suppl. 102, V:E (1968).
83. Friedman, L., and Friedman, M., "Effects of ions on vascular smooth muscle," in: Hamilton, W. F. (ed.), Handbook of Physiology, Section 2: Circulation, Vol. 2, Williams & Wilkins, Washington (1963), pp. 1135-1166.
84. Gabashvili, V. M., "The role of functional changes of the lumen of the major arteries of the brain in disturbances of the cerebral circulation," in: Maksudov, G. A. (ed.), Proceedings of a Symposium on the Pathogenesis of Transient Ischemia and Infarction of the Brain, Moscow (1968), pp. 64-72.
85. Gabashvili, V. M., and Mchedlishvili, G. I., "Reflex influences from the carotid sinus receptor zone on the internal carotid arteries," in: Vascular Diseases of the Brain, No. 2. Proceedings of the 4th All-Union Congress of Neuropathologists and Psychiatrists, Vol. 2, Moscow (1965), pp. 355-363.
86. Gaevskaya, M. S., Biochemistry of the Brain during the Process of Dying and Resuscitation, Moscow (1963) [Eng. trans.: Consultants Bureau, New York (1964)].
87. Gannushkina, I. V., "Aftereffects of closure of the intracerebral arteries and veins of the cerebral cortex," Zh. Nevropat. i Psikhiatr., 58(9):1025 (1958).
88. Gannushkina, I. V., "Aftereffects of closure of vessels of the cerebral cortex," Vopr. Neirokhir., No. 2, 1 (1959).
89. Gannushkina, I. V., and Shafranova, V. P., "Experimental data on the collateral circulation in vessels on the brain surface," Vopr. Neirokhir., No. 5, 13 (1963).
90. Garbulinskii, T., Gosk, A., and Mchedlishvili, G. I., "Photochemotachometric investigations of functions of the neuromuscular apparatus of the internal carotid arteries. Report 1. Experimental method and effects of certain physiologically active substances," Byull. Éksperim. Biol. i Med., 55(1):6 (1963).
91. Gedevanishvili, I. D., and Begiashvili, T. V., "Features of the vasodilator action of acetylcholine on peripheral arteries and arteriovenous anastomoses in the ear of the albino m mouse," Patol. Fiziol. i Éksper. Therap., 4(4):21, 1960.
92. Gerard, R. W., and Serota, H., "Localized thermal changes in brain," Amer. J. Physiol., 116:59 (1936).
93. Gindtse, B. M., The Arterial System of the Brain in Man and Animals, Part 1, Moscow (1946).
94. Goerttler, K., "Die funktionelle Bedeutung des Baues der Gefässwand," Dtsch. Z. Nervenheilk., 170:433 (1953).
95. Gotoh, F., Tazaki, Y., and Meyer, J. S., "Transport of gases through brain and their extravascular action," Exp. Neurol., 4:48 (1961).
96. Grach, S. N., Hurwitz, L. J., and McDowel, F., "Bilateral carotid occlusive disease," Arch. Neurol. (Chicago), 2:130 (1960).
97. Green, H. D., and Denison, A. B., "Absence of vasomotor responses to epinephrine in the isolated intracranial circulation," Circulat. Res., 4:565 (1956).
98. Gurfinkel', V. S., Meshalkin, E. N., Frantsev, V. I., and Golovanov, Yu. N., "Changes in the blood and cerebrospinal fluid pressure caused by disturbance of drainage by the system of the superior vena cava after cavopulmonary anastomosis," Abstracts of Proceedings of the 7th (Extended) Scientific Session on Cardiovascular Pathology at the M. D. Tsinamzgvrishvili Institute of Clinical and Experi-

mental Cardiology, Academy of Sciences of the Georgian SSR, Tbilisi (1961), pp. 248-249.

99. Gurvich, A. M., Shikunova, L. G., Novoderzhkina, I. S., and Bulanova, O. N., "The role of posthypoxic metabolic changes and cerebral edema in the recovery of central nervous system functions after full arrest of circulation," in: Mchedlishvili, G. I. (ed.), Correlation of Blood Supply with Metabolism and Function. Proceedings of an International Symposium (in Russian). Tbilisi (1969), pp. 233-243.

100. Häggendal, E., "Blood flow autoregulation of the cerebral gray matter with comments on its mechanism," in: Regional Cerebral Blood Flow. An International Symposium, Acta Neurol. Scand., Suppl. 14:104 (1965).

101. Häggendal, E., "Elimination of autoregulation during arterial and cerebral hypoxia," in: International Symposium on CBF and CSF., Scand. J. Lab. Clin. Invest., Suppl. 102, V̇-D (1968).

102. Häggendal, E., and Johansson, B., "Effects of arterial carbon dioxide tension and oxygen saturation on cerebral blood flow autoregulation in dogs," Acta Physiol. Scand., Suppl. 66, 258:27 (1965).

103. Handa, J., Meyer, J. S., Huber, P., and Yoshida, K., "Time course of development of cerebral collateral circulation," Vascular Dis., 2:271 (1965).

104. Harders, H., Über einige klinische Aspekte der intravasalen Erythrocytenballung," Schweiz. Med. Wschr., 87:11 (1957).

105. Harper, A. M., "Physiology of cerebral circulation," Brit. J. Anaesth., 37:225 (1965).

106. Harper, A. M. "The interrelationship between a_PCO_2 and blood pressure in the regulation of blood flow through the cerebral cortex," in: Regional Cerebral Blood Flow, Copenhagen (1965), pp. 94-103.

107. Harper, A. M., "Autoregulation of cerebral blood flow: influence of the arterial blood pressure on the blood flow through the cerebral cortex," J. Neurol. Neurosurg. Psychiat., 29:398 (1966).

108. Haynes, R. H., and Rodbard, S., "The system of arteries and arterioles: Biophysical principles and physiology," in: Abramson, D. (ed.), Blood Vessels and Lymphatics, Academic Press, New York–London (1962), pp. 25-40.

109. Hering, H. E., Die Karotissinusreflexe auf Herz und Gefässe, Dresden–Breslau, (1927).

110. Heymans, C., and Niel, E., Reflexogenic Areas of the Cardiovascular System, Little, London (1958).

111. Hill, L., The Physiology and Pathology of the Cerebral Circulation, London (1896).

112. Himwich, W. A., Knapp, F. M., Wenglarz, R. A., Martin, J. D., and Clark, M. E., "The circle of Willis as simulated by an engineering model," Arch. Neurol. (Chicago), 13:164 (1965).

113. Hirsch, H., Euler, K. H., and Schneider, M., "Über die Erholung und Wiederbelebung des Gehirns nach Ischämie bei Normothermie," Pflügers Arch. ges. Physiol., 265:281 (1957).

114. Hirsch, H., und Körner, K., "Über die Druck-Durchblutungs-Relation der Gehirngefässe," Pflügers Arch. ges. Physiol., 280:316 (1964).

115. Holmes, R. L., Newman, P. P., and Wolstencroft, J. H., "The distribution of carotid and vertebral blood in the brain of the cat," J. Physiol. (London), 140:236 (1958).

116. Holmqvist, B., Ingvar, D. H., and Sjesjö, B., "Cerebral sympathetic vasoconstriction and electroencephalogram," Acta Physiol. Scand., 40:146 (1957).

117. Huber, G. C., "Observations on the innervation of the intracranial vessels," J. Comp. Neurol., 9:1 (1899).

118. Hürthle, K., "Beiträge zur Hämodynamik. Dritte Abhandlung: Untersuchungen über die Innervation der Hirngefässe," Pflügers Arch. ges. Physiol., 44:561 (1899).

119. Hunter, W., "On the presence of nerve fibres in the cerebral vessels," J. Physiol. (London), 26:465 (1900-1901).

120. Ingvar, D. H., "Extraneuronal influence upon the electrical activity of isolated cortex following stimulation of the reticular formation," Acta Physiol. Scand., 33:169 (1955).

121. Ingvar, D. H., "Cortical state of excitability and cortical circulation," in: Reticular Formation of the Brain, Boston (1958), pp. 381-408.

122. Ingvar, D. H., Baldy-Moulinier, M., Sulg, I., and Hörman, S., "Regional cerebral blood flow related to EEG," in: Regional Cerebral Blood Flow. An International Symposium, Acta Neurol. Scand., Suppl., 14:179 (1965).

123. Ingvar, D. H., and Lassen, N. A., "Regional blood flow of the cerebral cortex determined by Krypton 85," Acta Physiol. Scand., 54:325 (1962).

124. Ingvar, D. H., Lübbers, D. W., and Sjesjö, B. K., "Normal and epileptic EEG patterns related to cortical oxygen tension in the cat,"

Acta Physiol. Scand., 55:210 (1962).

125. Ingvar, D., Mchedlishvili, G. I., and Ekberg, P., "Quantitative measurements of the local circulation in a cortical focus of paroxysmal activity," Dokl. Akad. Nauk SSSR, 166:1484 (1966).

126. Ingvar, D. H., Sjesjö, B., and Hertz, C. H., "Measurement of tissue pCO_2 in the brain," Experientia, 15:306 (1959).

127. Ingvar, D. H., and Söderberg, U., "A new method for measuring cerebral blood flow in relation to the electroencephalogram," Electroenceph. Clin. Neurophysiol., 8:403 (1956).

128. Iontov, A. S., "Sensory innervation of the cerebral arteries," Dokl. Akad. Nauk SSSR, 105:172 (1955).

129. Isenberg, I., "A note on the flow of blood in capillary tubes," Bull. Mathem. Biophys., 15:139 (1953).

130. Ivanov, On Nerve Endings in the Connective Tissue of Animals' Skin. Kazan' (1893). Cited in [148].

131. Iwoyama, T., Furness, J. B., and Burnstock, G., "Dual adrenergic and cholinergic innervation of the cerebral arteries of the rat. An ultrastructural study," Circulat. Res., 26:635 (1970).

132. Izmailova, I. V., "Evolution of the arterial system of the brain," Proceedings of the 5th All-Union Congress of Anatomists, Histologists, and Embryologists, Leningrad (1951), pp. 163-165.

133. Jackson, F. E., and Back, J. B., "Delayed arterial spasm and thrombosis as a cause of posttraumatic hemiplegia," Stroke, 1:278 (1970).

134. Jacobson, I., Harper, A. M., and McDowall, D. J., "Relationship between venous pressure and cortical blood flow," Nature, 200:173 (1963).

135. James, I. M., Millar, R. A., and Purves, M. J., "Observation on the extrinsic neural control of cerebral blood flow in the baboon," Circulat. Res., 25:77 (1969).

136. Kanzow, E., and Krause, D., "Vasomotorik der Hirnrinde und EEG–Aktivität wacher, frei beweglicher Katzen," Pflügers Arch. ges. Physiol., 274:447 (1962).

137. Kapustina, E. V., "Relationships between large arteries and veins in the pia mater of the cerebral hemispheres," Vopr. Neirokhir., No. 4, p. 13 (1953).

138. Kassil, G. N., Vein, A. M., and Kamenetskaya, B. N., "State of the blood-brain barrier during experimental exposure to various agents," Dokl. Akad. Nauk SSSR, 115:833 (1957).

139. Kedrov, A. A., Naumenko, A. I., and Degtyareva, Z. Ya., "Mechanism of the venous outflow from the skull," Byull. Éksperim. Biol. i Med., 38(9):10 (1954).

140. Kellie, G., Trans. Med.-Chir. Soc. Edinburgh, 1:84 (1824); ibid. 1:123 (1824). Cited in [111].

141. Kety, S. S., "Considerations of the effects of pharmacological agents on the over-all circulation and metabolism of the brain," in: Abramson, H. A. (ed.), Neuropharmacology, New York (1955), pp. 13-87.

142. Kety, S. S., "The cerebral circulation," in: McGoun, H. W. (ed.), Handbook of Physiology, Sect. 1, Neurophysiology, Vol. 3., Williams & Wilkins, Washington (1960), pp. 1751-1760.

143. Kety, S. S., and Schmidt, C. F., "The nitrous oxide method for the quantitative determination of cerebral blood flow in man: theory, procedure and normal values," J. Clin. Invest., 27:476 (1948).

144. Khayutin, V. M., "Effector structure and functional role of pressor reflexes," Vestn. Akad. Med. Nauk SSSR, No. 5, p. 70 (1961).

145. Kiss, F., and Tarjan, G., Hirnkreislauf und Schwangerschaftstoxikose, Leipzig (1959).

146. Klatzo, I., Miquel, J., and Otenasek, B., "The application of fluorescein labeled serum proteins (PLSP) to the study of vascular permeability in the brain," Acta Neuropathol., 2:144 (1962).

147. Klosovskii, B. N., "The capillary network of the brain in some pathological states of the central nervous system," Transactions of the Burdenko Institute of Neurosurgery, Vol. 1., Moscow (1948), pp. 21-44.

148. Klosovskii, B. N., The Circulation of Blood in the Brain, Moscow (1951).

149. Klosovskii, B. N., "The collateral circulation in the cortex and subcortical structures of the brain and occlusion of individual intracerebral arteries as a method of study of functions of the brain nuclei," in: Problems in the Physiology of the Central Nervous System, Moscow–Leningrad (1957), pp. 265-272.

150. Klosovskii, B. N., and Kosmarskaya, E. N., Active and Inhibitory States of the Brain, Moscow (1961).

151. Knisely, M. H., The Settling of Sludge during Life, Basel–New York (1961).

152. Knisely, M. H., Bloch, E. H., Eliot, T. S., and Warner, L., "Sludged blood," Science, 106:431 (1947).

153. Koch, E., Die Reflektorische Selbsteurung des Kreislaufes, Dresden–Leipzig (1931).
154. Konovalov, N. V., and Shmidt, E. V., "State and objects of scientific research in the field of vascular diseases of the nervous system and organization of their management," Zh. Nevropat. i Psikhiatr., 60:1557 (1960).
155. Konradi, G. P., "Peripheral mechanisms of the maintenance of vascular tone," in: Problems of Regulation of the Circulation, Moscow–Leningrad (1963), pp. 5-63.
156. Konradi, G. P., and Parolla, D. I., "Blood supply of the brain in various functional states," in: Symposium on "physiological Mechanisms of Regulation of the Cerebral Circulation," Leningrad (1963), pp. 72-119.
157. Konradi, G. P., and Parolla, D. I., "Peripheral tone and vasodilatation of cerebral vessels," Fiziol. Zh. SSSR, 52:1064 (1966).
158. Koreisha, L. A., "Analysis of the pathogenesis of disorders of the systemic and local circulation in clinical and experimental brain lesions," in: Disturbances of the Circulation in Brain Lesions, Moscow (1956), pp. 95-113.
159. Kosmarskaya, E. N., Volume, Conditions, and Sequelae of the Collateral Circulation in the Brain after Extra- and Intracranial Occlusion of the Main Arteries of the Brain, Dissertation, Moscow (1947).
160. Kosmarskaya, E. N., "The collateral circulation in the brain," Zh. Nevropat. i Psikhiatr., 53:702 (1953).
161. Kosmarskaya, E. N., and Kapustina, E. V., "Zones of collateral circulation in the brain," Byull. Éksperim. Biol. i Med., 35(4):78 (1952).
162. Kovács, A. G. R., Róheim, P. S., Iranyi, M., Cserhati, E., Gosztonyi, G., and Kovács, E., "Circulation and metabolism in the head of the dog in ischaemic shock," Acta. Physiol. Hung., 15:217 (1959).
163. Kowada, M., Ames, A., Majno, G., and Wright, L., "Cerebral ischemia. An improved experimental method for study; cardiovascular effects and demonstration of an early vascular lesion in the rabbit," J. Neurosurg., 28:150 (1968).
164. Koziner, V. B., "Features of the blood supply of the brain during replacement of blood loss by polyglucin and by blood," Patol. Fiziol. i Éksper. Terap., 9(1):11 (1965).
165. Koziner, V. B., and Kovalenko, E. A., "Oxygen tension in the brain tissues after acute blood loss and its treatment with blood substitutes," Patol. Fiziol. i Éksper. Terap., 8(1):56 (1964).
166. Krupp, P., Cerebrale Durchblutung und elektrische Hirnaktivität, Basel–New York (1966).
167. Krupp, P., and Carpi, A., "Die Beziehungen zwischen dem cerebrovasculären und elektrographischen Effekt der Hyperkapnie unter der Einwirkung von Barbituraten," Helv. Physiol. Acta, 22:C78 (1962).
168. Kukushkina, V. P., "Experimental investigations of the blood supply to the striatal system," Vopr. Neirokhir., No. 1, p. 14 (1956).
169. Kurusu, M., Fujita, B., Tanabe, T., Matsumata, H., Hatamochi, T., and Hiramoto, T., "On the regional peculiarity of the brain's circulatory response under various influences, especially of shock," Jap. Circulat. J., 21:264 (1957).
170. Lassen, N. A., "Cerebral blood flow and oxygen consumption in man," Physiol. Rev., 39:183 (1959).
171. Lassen, N. A. "Autoregulation of cerebral blood flow," Circulation Res., Vol. 15 Suppl. 1, pp. 201-204 (1964).
172. Lassen, N. A., "The adjustment of regional circulation to the local metabolic demand in the brain: breakdown of the 'metabolic control' following hypoxia," in: Mchedlishvili, G. I. (ed.), Correlation of Blood Supply with Metabolism and Function. Proceedings of an International Symposium, Tbilisi (1969), pp. 147-153.
173. Lavrent'ev, B. I., "Sensory innervation of the internal organs," in: Plechkova, E. K. (ed.), Morphology of the Sensory Innervation of the Internal Organs, Moscow (1947), pp. 5-21.
174. Lavrent'eva, N. B., Mchedlishvili, G. I., and Plechkova, E. K., "Distribution and activity of cholinesterase in the nervous structures of the pial arteries (a histochemical study)," Byull. Éxperim. Biol. i Med., 64(11):110 (1968).
175. Lazorthes, G., Vascularisation et Circulation Cérébrale, Paris (1961).
176. Legait, E., "Bourrelets valvulaires et bourrelets sphinctériens au niveau des artères cérébrales chez les vertébrés," Arch. Biol., 58:447 (1947).
177. Lende, R. A., "Local spasm in cerebral arteries," J. Neurosurg., 17:90 (1960).
178. Lerman, V. I., "The cerebral circulation in some vascular lesions and tumors of the brain," Author's Abstract of Doctoral Dissertation, Leningrad (1964).

179. Lerman, V. I., and Zlotnik, E. I., "Pressure in arteries of the cerebral cortex in hypotension produced by injection of ganglion-blocking drugs," Vopr. Neirokhir., No. 3, p. 7 (1959).
180. Levin, Yu. M., "Circulation in the head and brain after lethal blood loss and subsequent experimental resuscitation," Proceedings of the 4th Plenum of Pathophysiologists of Siberia and the Far East, Tomsk (1962), pp. 54-57.
181. Levin, Yu. M., The Regional Circulation after Lethal Blood Loss and Subsequent Resuscitation (Experimental Investigation), Author's Abstract of Doctoral Dissertation, Frunze (1965).
182. Levin, Yu. M., and Slovikov, B. I., "Oxygen tension and hemodynamics of the brain during lethal blood loss and subsequent resuscitation," Byull. Éksperim. Biol. i Med., 58(12):27, (1964).
183. Lierse, W., "Die Kapillardichte im Wirbeltiergehirn," Acta Anat., 54:1 (1963).
184. Lierse, W., "Gefässanordnung und Kapillardichte im Gehirn des Kaninchens," Acta Anat., 62:539 (1965).
185. Lierse, W., "Die postnatale Entwicklung der Kapillarisation im Gehirn der Maus," Acta Anat., 66:446 (1967).
186. Lierse, W., and Horstmann, E., "Quantitative anatomy of the cerebral vascular bed with special emphasis on homogeneity and inhomogeneity in small parts of the gray and white matter," in: Regional Cerebral Blood Flow. An International Symposium, Acta Neurol. Scand., Suppl. 14:15 (1965).
187. Lugovoi, L. A., "Circulation in individual areas of the cerebral cortex during photic and olfactory stimulation," Byull. Éksperim. Biol. i Med., 58(10):11 (1964).
188. Lurje, Z. G., "Pathogenesis of dynamic disturbances of the cerebral circulation," Zh. Nevropat. i Psikhiatr., 56(6):441 (1956).
189. Luse, S. A., "Ultrastructure of the brain and its relation to transport of metabolites," in: Ultrastructure and Metabolism of the Nervous System, Baltimore (1962), pp. 1-26.
190. Lutz, J., "Über veno-vasomotorische Gefässreaktionen im Mesenteriumkreislauf der Katze," Pflügers Arch. ges. Physiol., 287:330 (1966).
191. Lyubimova-Gerasimova, R. M., "Regulation of the cerebral circulation during exposure of the animal to ionizing radiation," Radiobiologiya, 2(1):82 (1962).
192. Lyakhovetskii, A. M., "Innervation of the dura mater," Arkh. Anat., Gistol., i Émbriol., 20(1):84 (1939).
193. Lyakhovetskii, A. M., "Innervation of the human pia mater," in: Plechkova, E. K. (ed.), Morphology of the Sensory Innervation of the Internal Organs, Moscow (1947), pp. 181-197.
194. Madzhagaladze, N. A., "Innervation of arteries of the head," Vopr. Neirokhir., No. 1, p. 26 (1960).
195. Magendie, F., Leçons sur les Phénomènes Physiques de la Vie, Vol. 3., Brussels (1838).
196. Maksimenkov, A. N., "Anatomical features of the structure of the venous system of the brain," in: Disturbances of the Circulation in Brain Lesions, Moscow (1956), pp. 228-240.
197. Mann, L. I., "Developmental aspects and the effect of carbon dioxide tension on fetal cephalic blood flow," Exp. Neurol., 26:136 (1970).
198. Marshak, M. E., "Principles governing regulation of the region circulation," Vestn. Akad. Med. Nauk SSSR, No. 9, 36 (1959).
199. Marshak, M. E., "Regulation of the regional circulation," in: Current Problems in the Physiology and Pathology of the Circulation, Moscow (1961), pp. 166-192.
200. Marshak, M. E., Physiological Significance of Carbon Dioxide, Moscow (1969).
201. Marshak, M. E., Sanotskaya, N. V., and Ryzhova, N. M., "On factors affecting the regional and zonal oxygen tension in tissue," in: Mchedlishvili, G. I. (ed.), Correlation of Blood Supply with Metabolism and Function. Proceedings of an International Symposium, Tbilisi (1969), pp. 101-109.
202. McDonald, D. A., and Potter, J. M., "The distribution of blood to the brain," J. Physiol. (London) 114:356 (1951).
203. McDowall, D. G., and Harper, A. M., "The relationship between blood flow and the extracellular pH of the cerebral cortex," in: Bain, H., and Harper, A. M. (eds.), Blood Flow through Organs and Tissues, Edinburgh and London (1968), pp. 261-278.
204. Mchedlishvili, G. I., "Investigations of the mechanism of capillary stasis," Transactions of the Institute of Physiology, Academy of Sciences of the Georgian SSR, Vol. 9. Tbilisi (1953), pp. 279-292.
205. Mchedlishvili, G. I., "New experimental data on changes in the capillary circulation," Soobshch. Akad. Nauk Gruz. SSR, 17:537 (1956).
206. Mchedlishvili, G. I., "Methods of studying the capillary circulation in the cerebral cortex,"

in: Current Problems in the Physiology of the Nervous and Muscular Systems, Dedicated to Academician I. S. Beritashvili, Tbilisi (1956), pp. 549-554.

207. Mchedlishvili, G. I., "The extracerebral mechanism of regulation of the cerebral circulation," in: Abstracts of Proceedings of the 17th Scientific Session of the Division of Medical and Biological Sciences, Academy of Sciences of the Georgian SSR, Tbilisi (1957), pp. 9-12.

208. Mchedlishvili, G. I., Capillary Circulation, Tbilisi (1958).

209. Mchedlishvili, G. I., "Role of the internal carotid and vertebral arteries in regulation of the cerebral circulation," Fiziol. Zh. SSSR, 45:1221 (1959).

210. Mchedlishvili, G. I., "Investigations into the localization of 'closing mechanisms' on regional brain arters (internal carotid and vertebral arteries)," Dokl. Akad. Nauk SSSR, 124:1371 (1959).

211. Mchedlishvili, G. I., "The action of adrenalin on the regional arteries of the brain," Byull. Éksperim. Biol. i Med., 49(5):10 (1960).

212. Mchedlishvili, G. I., "On the independence of mechanisms regulating the lumen of regional arteries of the brain (the internal carotid and vertebral arteries) and of the pial arteries," Byull. Éksperim. Biol. i Med., 49(6):21 (1960).

213. Mchedlishvili, G. I., "Physiological mechanisms of the cerebral circulation in terminal states," Fiziol. Zh. SSSR, 46:1210 (1960).

214. Mchedlishvili, G. I., "Changes in the cerebral circulation during resuscitation by intra-arterial blood transfusion," Patol. Fiziol. i Éksper. Terap., 4(4):14 (1960).

215. Mchedlishvili, G. I., "Investigations of mechanisms of regulation of the cerebral circulation. Report 1. Regional arteries of the brain as regulators of inflow of blood into the brain," Transactions of the Institute of Physiology, Academy of Sciences of the Georgian SSR, Vol. 12, Tbilisi (1961), pp. 121-136.

216. Mchedlishvili, G. I., "Investigations of the cerebral vessels and circulation by intravital fixation of the tissues," Transactions of the Institute of Experimental Morphology, Academy of Sciences of the Georgian SSR, Vol. 9, Tbilisi (1961), pp. 121-127.

217. Mchedlishvili, G. I., "A thorax–head preparation for investigation of the cerebral circulation," Byull. Éksperim. Biol. i Med., 53(2): 123 (1962).

218. Mchedlishvili, G. I., "Mechanisms of regulation of the cerebral circulation. Report 2. Functional differences between various parts of the arterial system of the brain," Transactions of the Institute of Physiology, Academy of Sciences of the Georgian SSR, Vol. 13, Tbilisi (1963).

219. Mchedlishvili, G. I., "The use of differential manometry (in particular, of Huerthle's method) for investigating the cerebral circulation," Patol. Fiziol. i Éksper. Terap., 7(3):75 (1963).

220. Mchedlishvili, G. I., "The functional role of different parts of the vascular system of the brain," in: Metabolismus Parietis Vasorum, Prague (1963), pp. 364-369.

221. Mchedlishvili, G. I., "Functional constriction of the system of regional arteries of the brain (internal carotid and vertebral arteries) as a cause of cerebrovascular disturbances," Zh. Nevropat. i Psikhiatr., 64(5):663 (1964).

222. Mchedlishvili, G. I., "Vascular mechanisms pertaining to the intrinsic regulation of the cerebral circulation," Circulation, 30:597 (1964).

223. Mchedlishvili, G. I., Function of the Vascular Mechanisms of the Brain, Leningrad (1968).

224. Mchedlishvili, G. I., "The spasm of the internal carotid arteries," in: Brock, M. et al. (eds.), Cerebral Blood Flow, Berlin–Heidelberg–New York (1969), pp. 98-100.

225. Mchedlishvili, G. I., "The conjectural role of the Fahraeus–Lindqvist rheological phenomenon in some microcirculatory events," in: Harders, H. (ed.), 5th European Conference on Microcirculation, Bibl. Anat. No. 10, Basel–New York (1969), pp. 66-73.

226. Mchedlishvili, G. I., "Distribution of blood and its constituents in the microcirculation system," Vestn. Armyan. SSR, No. 11, p.48 (1970).

227. Mchedlishvili, G. I., and Akhobadze, V. A., "Dynamics of changes in the cerebral circulation in traumatic edema of the brain," Vopr. Neirokhir., No. 2, p. 13 (1960).

228. Mchedlishvili, G. I., and Akhobadze, V. A., "The cerebral arterial system in brain injury and during traumatic edema," Physiol. Bohemoslov., 10:8 (1961).

229. Mchedlishvili, G. I., and Akhobadze, V. A., "The functional state of the capillary and venous systems of the brain in cerebral traumatic edema," Physiol. Bohemoslov., 10:15 (1961).

230. Mchedlishvili, G. I., and Akhobadze, V. A., "Elevation of the intracranial pressure and deficiency of blood supply to the brain," Pro-

ceedings of a Joint Scientific Session of Transcaucasian Institutes of the Academy of Medical Sciences of the USSR on Cardiovascular Pathology, Tbilisi (1964), pp. 313-315.

231. Mchedlishvili, G. I., Akhobadze, V. A., and Ormotsadze, L. G., "Dynamics of cerebrovascular disorders and their compensation during temporary occlusion of the aorta," Patol. Fiziol. i Éksper. Terap., 6(3):17 (1962).

232. Mchedlishvili, G. I., Akhobadze, V. A., and Ormotsadze, L. G., "Hemodynamic mechanisms of compensation of the cerebral circulation during temporary occlusion of the cranial (superior) vena cava," Fiziol. Zh. SSSR, 48:684 (1962).

233. Mchedlishvili, G. I., Amashukeli, G. V., Antia, R. V., Dolidze, V. A., Kolelishvili, R. I., Mitagvaria, N. P., and Nikolaishvili, L. S., "Polygraphic studies of different parameters of blood supply, metabolism and activity of the brain under conditions of terminal state and subsequent resuscitation," in: Negovskii, V. A., and Gurvich, A. M. (eds.), Period of Recovery after Reanimation, Moscow (1970), pp. 73-81.

234. Mchedlishvili, G. I., and Baramadze, D. G., "Functional behavior of the small arteries of the cerebral cortex," Dokl. Akad. Nauk SSSR, 163:529 (1965).

235. Mchedlishvili, G. I., and Baramidze, D. G., "The functional behavior of cortical blood vessels under conditions of convulsive activity," Byull. Éxperim. Biol. i. Med., 64(11):74 (1967).

236. Mchedlishvili, G. I., and Baramidze, D. G., "Functional behavior of the precortical arteries under conditions of experimental hypo- and hypertension," Byull. Éxper. Biol. i Med., in press.

237. Mchedlishvili, G. I., Baramidze, D. G., and Nikolaishvili, L. S., "Functional behavior of the pial and cortical arteries in conditions of increased metabolic demand from the cerebral cortex," Nature, 213:506 (1967).

238. Mchedlishvili, G. I., Baramidze, D. G., Nikolaishvili, L. S., and Ormotsadze, L. G., "The function of the vascular mechanisms of the brain in the regulation of the adequate blood supply to the cerebral cortex," in: Mchedlishvili, G. I. (ed.), Correlation of Blood Supply with Metabolism and Function. Proceedings of an International Symposium, Tbilisi (1969), pp. 85-100.

239. Mchedlishvili, G. I., and Devdariani, M. G., "Investigations of mechanisms of compensatory reactions of the cerebral arteries during their occlusion," Proceedings of the Second Transcaucasian Conference of Pathophysiologists on Defensive and Adaptive Reactions of the Organism, Erevan (1962), pp. 251-252.

240. Mchedlishvili, G. I., and Devdariani, M. G., "Intrinsic mechanisms determining the collateral circulation in the brain," Patol. Fiziol. i Éksper. Terap., 8(3):20 (1964).

241. Mchedlishvili, G. I., and Gabashvili, V. M., "Investigation of the genesis of pathological constriction and spasm of the internal carotid arteries," Patol. Fiziol. i Éksper. Terap., 9(6):9 (1965).

242. Mchedlishvili, G. I., Garbuliński, T., and Gosk, A., "Researches on functions of the internal carotid arteries," Acta Physiol. Polonica, 13:695 (1962).

243. Mchedlishvili, G. I., Garbulińskii, T., and Gosk, A., "Photohemotachometric investigations of the neuromuscular apparatus of the internal carotid arteries. Report 2. Control by the sympathetic nervous system," Byull. Éksperim. Biol. i Med., 55(2):17 (1963).

244. Mchedlishvili, G. I., Ingvar, D. H., Baramidze, D. G., and Eckberg, R., "Blood flow and vascular behavior in the cerebral cortex related to strychnine-induced spike activity," Exp. Neurol., 26:411 (1970).

245. Mchedlishvili, G. I., Kaufman, O. Ya., Ormotsadze, L. G., and Borodula, V. A., "Functional-morphological studies of the spasm of the internal carotid artery," Krovoobrashchenie (Erevan), in press.

246. Mchedlishvili, G. I., Kometiani, P. A., and Ormotsadze, L. G., "Involvement of calcium ions in the formation of vascular tone and in the serotonin vasoconstrictor effect on the internal carotid artery," Byull Éxperim. Biol. i Med., in press.

247. Mchedlishvili, G. I., Kuparadze, M. R., and Baramidze, D. G., "Dynamics of changes in vessels of the cerebral cortex during the development of postischemic edema," Byull. Éksperim. Biol. i Med., 60(12):30 (1965).

248. Mchedlishvili, G. I., Mitagvaria, N. P., and Ormotsadze, L. G., "Computation of the resistance in larger and smaller arteries of the brain with a mathematical model," Fiziol. Zh. SSSR, 57:575 (1971).

249. Mchedlishvili, G. I., and Nikolaishvili, L. S., "The nervous mechanism of nutritive reactions of the pial arteries supplying blood to the cerebral cortex," Dokl. Akad. Nauk SSSR, 156:968 (1964).

250. Mchedlishvili, G. I., and Nikolaishvili, L. S., "Investigations of the physiological mechanisms of correlation between the blood supply and functional state of the cerebral cortex," Fiziol. Zh. SSSR, 52:380 (1966).
251. Mchedlishvili, G. I., and Nikolaishvili, L. S., "Zum nervösen Mechanismus der funktionellen Dilatation der Piaarterien," Pflügers Arch. ges. Physiol., 296:14 (1967).
252. Mchedlishvili, G. I., and Nikolaishvili, L. S., "Evidence of a cholinergic nervous mechanism mediating the autoregulatory dilatation of the cerebral blood vessels," Pflügers Arch. ges. Physiol., 315:27 (1970).
253. Mchedlishvili, G. I., Nikolaishvili, L. S., Antia, R. V., Mitagvaria, N. P., and Baramidze, D. G., "The physiological mechanism of dilatation of the pial arteries in response to a reduced systemic arterial pressure," Fiziol. Zh. SSSR, 56:240 (1971).
254. Mchedlishvili, G. I., and Ormotsadze, L. G., "Investigations of reflex effects from the venous sinuses on regional arteries of the brain," Byull. Éksperim. Biol. i Med., 53(2):9 (1962).
255. Mchedlishvili, G. I., and Ormotsadze, L. G., "A hemodynamic mechanism compensating for decreased blood supply to the cerebral cortex," Physiol. Bohemoslov, 12:100 (1963).
256. Mchedlishvili, G. I., and Ormotsadze, L. G., "A new modification of resistography of the *in situ* isolated internal carotid artery for investigation of the vascular spasm," Patol. Fiziol. i Éxper. Terap., 13(3):72 (1970).
257. Mchedlishvili, G. I., Ormotsadze, L. G., and Amashukeli, G. V., "Resistography of the isolated internal carotid artery," Byull. Éksperim. Biol. i Med., 64(10):3 (1967).
258. Mchedlishvili, G. I., Ormotsadze, L. G., and Kometiani, P. A., "The serotonin effect on the *in situ* isolated internal carotid artery," Patol. Fiziol. i Éxper. Terap., in press.
259. Mchedlishvili, G. I., Ormotsadze, L. G., Nicolaishvili, L. S., and Baramidze, D. G., "Reaction of different parts of the cerebral vascular system in asphyxia," Exp. Neurol., 18:239 (1967).
260. Mchedlishvili, G. I., Ormotsadze, L. G., Samvelian, V. M., and Amashukeli, G. V., "Cholinergic and adrenergic receptors in the walls of the internal carotid arteries," Dokl. Akad. Nauk SSSR, 184:999 (1969).
261. Mercker, H., and Schneider, M., "Über Capillarenveränderungen des Gehirns bei Höhenanpassung," Pflügers Arch. ges. Physiol., 251:49 (1949).
262. Meyer, J. S., "Circulatory changes following occlusion of the middle cerebral artery and their relation to function," J. Neurosurg., 15:653 (1958).
263. Meyer, J. S., and Denny-Brown, D., "Studies of cerebral circulation in brain injury. I. Validity of combined local cerebral electropolarography, thermometry and steady potentials as an indicator of local circulatory and functional changes," Electroenceph. Clin. Neurophysiol., 7:511 (1955).
264. Meyer, J. S., and Gotoh, F., "Interaction of cerebral hemodynamics and metabolism," Neurology, 11(2):46 (1961).
265. Meyer, J. S., Gotoh, F., and Favale, E., "Effects of carotid compression on cerebral metabolism and electroencephalogram," Electroenceph. Clin. Neurophysiol., 19:362 (1965).
266. Meyer, J. S., Gotoh, F., Tazaki, Y., Hamaguchi, K., Ishikawa, S., Nouaihat, F., and Symon, L., "Regional cerebral blood flow and metabolism *in vivo*," Arch. Neurol., 7:560 (1962).
267. Meyer, J. S., Kondo, A., Nomura, F., Sakamoto, K., and Taraura, T., "Cerebral hemodynamics and metabolism following experimental head injury," J. Neurosurg., 32:303 (1970).
268. Meyer, J. S., Nomura, F., Sakamoto, K., and Kondo, A., "Effect of stimulation of the brainstem reticular formation on cerebral blood flow and oxygen consumption," Electroenceph. Clin. Neurophysiol., 26:125 (1969).
269. Meyer, J. S., and Portnoy, H., "Post-epileptic paralysis. A clinical and experimental study," Brain, 82:162 (1959).
270. Meyer, J. S., and Waltz, A. C., "Effects of changes in composition of plasma on blood flow. I. Lipids and lipid fractions," Neurology, 9:728 (1959).
271. Meyer, J. S., Waltz, A. C., and Gotoh, F., "Pathogenesis of cerebral vasospasm in hypertensive encephalopathy. I. Effects of acute increases in intraluminal pressure on pial blood flow," Neurology 10:735 (1960).
272. Meyer, J. S., Yoshida, K., and Sakamoto, K., "Autonomic control of cerebral blood flow measured by electromagnetic flowmeters," Neurology, 17:638 (1967).
273. Mikhailov, S. S., "Structural features of the cavernous sinus," in: Disturbances of the Circulation in Brain Lesions, Moscow (1956), pp. 254-263.

274. Mikhailov, S. S., "The nervous apparatus of the cavernous venous sinus," Arkh. Anat., Gistol., i Embriol., 41(10):61 (1961).

275. Mikhailov, S. S., "Reflex reactions of the blood pressure and respiration to stimulation of the cavernous venous sinus," Fiziol. Zh. SSSR, 49:822 (1963).

276. Mitagvaria, N. P., "An adequate mathematical model of interrelationship of basic hemodynamic parameters of the brain," Soobshch. Akad. Nauk Gruz.SSR, 60:697 (1970).

277. Molnár, A., Sur le Contrôle Nerveux de la Circulation Sanguine Regionale des Centres Cérébraux, Budapest (1967).

278. Monro, A., Observation on the Structure and Function of the Nervous System, Edinburgh (1783), Cited in [111].

279. Moskalenko, Yu. E., Dynamics of the Brain Blood Volume under Normal Conditions and Gravitational Stresses, Leningrad (1967).

280. Moskalenko, Yu. E., Demchenko, I. T., Savich, A. A., and Weinstein, G. P., "Peculiarities of the correlation between blood flow and some indices of functional activity in circumscribed brain regions," in: Mchedlishvili, G. I. (ed.), Correlation of Blood Supply with Metabolism and Function. Proceedings of an International Symposium, Tbilisi (1969), pp. 154-166.

281. Moskalenko, Yu. E., and Filanovskaya, T. P., "On changes in pulsatile blood flow in arteries of the cranial base," Fiziol. Zh. SSSR, 53:1387 (1967).

282. Moskalenko, Yu. E., and Naumenko, A. I., Hemodynamics of cerebral circulation," in: Simonson, E. (ed.), Cerebral Ischemia, Thomas, Springfield (1964), pp. 21-61.

283. Nadareishvili, K. Sh., "Fluctuations in tone of regional arteries of the brain synchronized with respiration," in: Mchedlishvili, G. I. (ed.), Current problems in Morphology, Physiology, and Pathology, Dedicated to V. V. Voronin, Tbilisi (1962), pp. 135-142.

284. Nadareishvili, K. Sh,. "Direct reactions of the cardiovascular system of animals to the external action of ionizing radiation," Trud. Inst. Fiziol. Akad. Nauk Gruz., SSR 13:219 (1963).

285. Naumenko, A. I., "The physiological mechanisms of regulation of the cerebral circulation," in: Kedrov, A. A. (ed.), Problems of Physiology of the Cerebral Circulation, Leningrad (1970), pp. 76-105.

286. Naumenko, A. I., Antonov, A. K., Moskalenko, Yu. E., and Sazonov, S. Ya., "New data concerning the mechanism of the intracranial circulation," Fiziol. Zh. SSSR, 48:1251 (1962).

287. Negovskii, V. A., The Pathophysiology and Treatment of Agony and Clinical Death, Moscow (1954).

288. Nelson, E., and Rennals, M., "Electron microscopic studies on intracranial vascular nerves in the cat," Scand. Lab. Clin. Invest., Suppl. 102, VI:A (1968).

289. Ngai, E. H., and Nelson, E. C., "Effect of induced hypotension on carotid portion of cerebral blood flow," J. Appl. Physiol., 7:176 (1954).

290. Nielsen, K. C., and Owman, Ch., "Adrenergic innervation of pial arteries related to the circle of Willis in the cat," Brain Res., 6:773 (1967).

291. Nikolaishvili, L. S., "On the effect of carbon dioxide on the pial arteries which supply blood to the cerebral cortex," Soobshch. Akad. Nauk Gruz.SSR, 46:483 (1967).

292. Noguchi, T., Mori, A., and Shimazono, Y., "An experimental study on the correlation between electrical activity and cerebral blood flow in convulsive processes," Epilepsia, 1:208 (1959).

293. Novoderzhkina, I. S., "The role of edema of the brain during the restoration of neurological functions in revival following mechanical asphyxia," Patol. Fiziol. i. Éxper. Terap., 13(6):72 (1969).

294. Nozhnikov, A., On the Structure of Cerebral Arteries and Meninges, Kharkov (1899).

295. Ognev, B. V. (ed.), The Blood Supply of the Central and Peripheral Nervous System in Man, Moscow (1950).

296. Opdyke, D. F., "Circulatory effects of partial cerebral ischemia," Amer. J. Physiol., 146:467 (1946).

297. Oppel, V. A., Course of Clinical Lectures on Special Surgery, Moscow–Leningrad (1930).

298. Orestenko, Yu., "Changes in blood supply and temperature of the brain associated with dura mater stimulation or local extirpation of brain tissue," Fiziol. Zh. SSSR, 51:1043 (1965).

299. Ormotsadze, L. G., "Elucidation of the closing mechanisms of the major arteries of the amphibian brain," Soobshch. Akad. Nauk Gruz.SSR, 55:685 (1969).

300. Ormotsadze, L. G., Samvelian, V. M., Nikolaishvili, L. S., and Mchedlishvili, G. I., "The

effect of serotonin on internal carotid and pial arteries," Krovoobrashchenie (Erevan), 2(4): 16 (1969).

301. Owman, C., Falck, B., and Mchedlishvili, G. I., "Adrenergic structures of the pial arteries and their connections with the cerebral cortex," Byull. Éksperim. Biol. i Med., 59(6):98 (1965).

302. Parin, V. V., and Mchedlishvili, G. I., "Progress and objects of microcirculation research," Vestn. Akad. Med. Nauk SSSR, No. 6, p. 3 (1964).

303. Parolla, D. I., "Effect of stimulation of afferent fibers of somatic nerves on the blood flow in the brain," in: Problems in Regulation of the Circulation, Moscow–Leningrad (1963), pp. 133-151.

304. Pease, D. C., "Microscopic and submicroscopic anatomy," in: Abramson, D. I. (ed.), Blood Vessels and Lymphatics, Academic Press, New York–London (1962), pp. 12-25.

305. Pease, D. C., and Schultz, R. L., "Circulation to the brain and spinal cord. Submicroscopical anatomy," in: Abramson, D. I. (ed.), Blood Vessels and Lymphatics, Academic Press, New York–London (1962), pp. 233-239.

306. Penfield, W., "Intracerebral vascular nerves," Arch. Neurol. Psychiat. (Chicago), 27:30 (1932).

307. Perli, P. D., and Konovalova, M. K., "Influence of the carotid sinus on the cerebral circulation," Transactions of the Institute of Experimental and Clinical Medicine, Academy of Sciences of the Latvian SSR, Vol. 24, Riga (1961), pp. 141-147.

308. Pfeifer, R. A., Die angioarchitektonische areale Gliederung der Grosshirnrinde auf Grund vollkommener Gefässinjektionspräparate vom Gehirn des Macacus Rhesus dargestellt, Leipzig (1940).

309. Piotrovich, A. S., "Effect of stimulation of mechanoreceptors of the spleen on some indices of the cerebral circulation," in: Pathogenesis, Clinical Features, Treatment, and Prevention of the Most Important Diseases, Volgograd (1963), pp. 141-143.

310. Piotrovich, A. S., "Effect of stimulation of mechanoreceptors of the spleen on some indices of the cerebral circulation," Byull. Éksperim. Biol. i Med., 59(1):3 (1965).

311. Plechkova, E. K., Mchedlishvili, G. I., Lavrent'eva, N. B., and Nikolaishvili, L. S., "On the cholinergic mechanism responsible for functional dilatation of the arteries supplying the cerebral cortex," in: Mchedlishvili, G. I. (ed.), Correlation of Blood Supply with Metabolism and function. Proceedings of an International Symposium, Tbilisi (1969), pp. 172-184.

312. Pokrovskaya, G. A., "On nerve cells and ganglia in the internal carotid nerve," Vestn. Leningrad. Univ., No. 9, p. 103 (1958).

313. Pool, J. L., "Vasocardiac effects of the circle of Willis," Arch. Neurol. Psychiat. (Chicago), 78:355 (1957).

314. Poole, E. W., "Reactions of the cat pial circulation to hypotensive states induced by hexamethonium bromide," Arch. Neurol. Psychiat. (Chicago), 71:640 (1954).

315. Potter, J. M., "Redistribution of blood to the brain due to localised cerebral arterial spasm. I. The possible importance of the small peripheral anastomotic cerebral arteries," Brain, 82:367 (1959).

316. Prados, M., Strowger, B., and Feindel, W. H., "Studies on cerebral edema. I. Reaction of the brain to air exposure; pathologic changes," Arch. Neurol. Psychiat. (Chicago), 54:163 (1945).

317. Pratusevich, Yu. M., "Study of chronic mental overstrain according to the data of brain blood circulation," in: Palladin, A. V., and Kometiani, P. A. (eds.), Proceedings of the Fifth All-Union Neurochemical Conference, Tbilisi (1970), pp. 501-506.

318. Rapella, C. E., and Green, H. D., "Autoregulation of canine cerebral blood flow," Circulat. Res., Vol. 15 Suppl. 1, p. 205 (1964).

319. Raynor, R. B., and McMurtry, J. G., "Prevention of serotonin-produced cerebral vasospasm," J. Neurosurg., 20:94 (1963).

320. Raynor, R. B., and Ross, G., "Arteriography and vasospasm. The effect of intracranial contrast media on vasospasm," J. Neurosurg., 17:1055 (1960).

321. Reichel, K., and Kanzow, E., "Der Einfluss von Barbiturat-Narkose und CO_2 auf die Autoregulation der Hirnrindendurchblutung," Pflügers Arch, ges. Physiol., 279:R14 (1964).

322. Rein, H., "Uber Besonderheiten der Blutzirkulation in der Arteria carotis," Z. Biol., 89:307 (1929).

323. Rein, H., "Vasomotorische Regulationen," Ergebn. Physiol., 32:28 (1931).

324. Reivich, M., "Arterial pCO_2 and cerebral hemodynamics," Amer. J. Physiol., 206:25 (1964).

325. Reivich, M., Marshall, W. J. S., and Kessel, N., "Loss of autoregulation produced by cerebral trauma," in: Brock, M. et al. (eds.), Cerebral Blood Flow. Berlin–Heidelberg–New York (1969), pp. 205-208.

326. Riggs, H. E., and Griffiths, J. O., "Anomalies of the circle of Willis in persons with nervous and mental diseases," Arch. Neurol. Psychiat. (Chicago), 39:1353 (1938).
327. Rodbard, S., and Saiki, H., "Mechanism of the pressure response to increased intracranial pressure," Amer. J. Physiol., 168:234 (1952).
328. Rodbard, S., and Stone, W., "Pressor mechanisms induced by intracranial compression," Circulation, 12:883 (1955).
329. Romanova, N. P., "Dynamics of histopathological changes in the brain in experimental hypoxia," Zh. Nevropat. i Psikhiatr., 56(1):49 (1956).
330. Rosenblum, W. I., and Zweifach, B. W., "Cerebral microcirculation in the mouse brain," Neurology, 9:414 (1963).
331. Rothernberg, S. F., and Corday, E., "Etiology of the transient cerebral stroke," J. Amer. Med. Assn., 164:2005 (1957).
332. Rothernberg, S. F., and Corday, E., "Primary and traumatic cerebral angiospasm," in: Meyer, J. S., and Gastaut, H. (eds.), Cerebral Anoxia and Electroencephalogram, Thomas, Springfield (1961), pp. 130-133.
333. Roy, C. S., and Sherrington, C. S., "The regulation of the blood supply of the brain," J. Physiol. (London), 11:85 (1890).
334. Ryzhova, N. M., "Reflex effects on the cerebral circulation. Report 1. Blood supply to the brain during stimulation of interoceptors of the small intestine," Byull. Éksperim. Biol. i Med., 43(2):13 (1957).
335. Ryzhova, N. M., "The cerebral circulation in hypotension produced by compression of both carotid arteries," in: Problems in General and Age Physiology and Pathology. Tr. Inst. Normalnoi i Patol. Fiziol. Akad. Med. Nauk SSSR, 3:32 (1959).
336. Ryzhova, N. M., "Mechanism of carbon dioxide effect on cerebral vessels," Fiziol. Zh. SSSR, 52:1079 (1966).
337. Sagawa, Kiichi, and Guyton, A. C., "Pressure-flow relationships in isolated canine cerebral circulation," Amer. J. Physiol., 200:711 (1961).
338. Saradzhishvili, P. M., and Muskhelishvili, S. V., "Relationship between the carotid sinus reflex and the cerebral circulation," Collection of Papers to Commemorate 50 Years of Scientific and Teaching Activity of V. V. Voronin, Tbilisi (1941), pp. 232-237.
339. Scharrer, E., "Capillaries and mitochondria in neuropil," J. Comp. Neurol., 83:237 (1945).
340. Scheinberg, P., and Joyne, H. W., "Factors influencing cerebral blood flow and metabolism," Circulation, 5:225 (1952).
341. Schmidt, C. F., The Cerebral Circulation in Health and Disease, Thomas, Springfield (1950).
342. Schmidt, H. W., "Mikroskopische Lebensbeobachtungen an den Hirngefässen unter physiologischen und pathologischen Bedingungen," in: Europäische Konferenz über Mikrozirkulation., Bibl. Anat., Vol. 1., Hamburg (1961), pp. 182-190.
343. Schneider, M., "The metabolism of the brain in ischaemia and hypothermia," in: Richter, D. (ed.), Metabolism of the Nervous System, Pergamon, New York–London (1957), pp. 238-244.
344. Schneider, M., "Brain circulation and revival after ischemia with remarks on the problem of vasospasm in the brain," J. Med. Libanais, 12:18 (1959).
345. Schneider, M., Physiologic des Menschen, Berlin–Göttingen–Heidelberg (1964).
346. Schneider, M., Überlebens- und Wiederbelebungszeit von Gehirn, Herz, Leber, Niere nach Ischaemie und Anoxie, Köln und Opladen (1965).
347. Schneider, M., and Schneider, D., "Untersuchungen über die Regulierung der Gehirndurchblutung. III. Mitteilung: Die Rolle des Carotissinus bei der Regulierung der Gehirndurchblutung," Arch. Exp. Path. Pharmak., 176:393 (1935).
348. Schultz, A., "Zur Lehre von der Blutbewegung im Innern des Schädels," St. Petersburger Med. Ztschr., 11(2):122 (1866).
349. Serota, H. M., and Gerard, R. W., "Localized thermal changes in the cat's brain," J. Neurophysiol., 1:115 (1938).
350. Severinghaus, J. W., "Special summary presented at the end of the Symposium," in: International Symposium on CSF and CBF., Scand. J. Lab. Clin. Invest., Suppl. 102, VIII:K (1968).
351. Severinghaus, J. W., "International Symposium on CSF and CBF," Anaesthesia, 29:1232 (1968).
352. Shalit, M. N., Reinmuth, O., Shimojyo, S., Lockhart, W., and Scheinberg, P., "The mechanism of action of CO_2 in the regulation of cerebral blood flow," in: Bain, H. and Harper, A. M. (eds.), Blood Flow through Organs and Tissues, Edinburgh and London (1968), pp. 279-281.
353. Shalit, M. N., Shimojyo, S., and Reinmuth, O. M., "Carbon dioxide and cerebral circulatory

control. I. The extravascular effect," Arch. Neurol. (Chicago), 17:298 (1967).

354. Shenkin, H. A., Cabieses, F., van den Noordt, G., et al., "Symposium on intracranial vascular abnormalities; hemodynamic effect of unilateral carotid ligation on cerebral circulation in man," J. Neurosurg., 8:38 (1951).

355. Shenkin, H. A., and Novack, P., "Clinical implications of recent studies on cerebral circulation," Arch. Neurol. Psychiat. (Chicago), 71:148 (1954).

356. Shimizu, T., "Experimental study of cerebral circulation," J. Kyoto Pref. Med. Univ., 63: 603 (1958).

357. Shmidt, E. V., Stenosis and Thrombosis of the Carotid Arteries and Disturbances of the Cerebral Circulation, Moscow (1963).

358. Sjesjö, B. K., "A method for continuous measurement of the carbon dioxide tension in the cerebral cortex," Acta Physiol. Scand., 51:297 (1961).

359. Slovikov, B. I., "Oxygen tension in the brain and liver during lethal blood loss and subsequent resuscitation after clinical death," Proceedings of the 4th Plenum of Pathophysiologists of Siberia and the Far East, Tomsk (1962), pp. 57-60.

360. Smirnov, L. I., Special Pathological Anatomy of Brain Trauma Uncomplicated by Infection. Pathological Anatomy and Pathogenesis of Traumatic Diseases of the Nervous System, Part 2, Moscow (1949).

361. Söderberg, U., "A new technique of recording cortical blood flow in cats, suitable for measurment of arterio-venous concentration differences," Experientia, 13:343 (1962).

362. Söderberg, U., "Neurophysiological aspects of homeostasis," Ann. Rev. Physiol., 26:271 (1964).

363. Söderberg, U., and Weckman, N., "Changes in cerebral blood supply caused by changes in the pressure drop along arteries to the brain of the cat," Experientia, 15:346 (1959).

364. Sokoloff, L., "The action of drugs on the cerebral circulation," Pharmacol. Rev., 11:1 (1959).

365. Sokoloff, L., "Metabolism of the central nervous system *in vivo*, " in: McGoun, H. W. (ed.), in: Handbook of Physiology, Sect. 1, Neurophysiology, Vol. 3., Williams and Wilkins, Washington (1960), pp. 1843-1864.

366. Sokoloff, L., "Local cerebral circulation at rest and during altered cerebral activity induced by anesthesia or visual stimulation," in: Kety, S. S., and Elkes, J. (eds.), Regional Neurochemistry, Pergamon, Oxford (1961), pp. 107-117.

367. Sokoloff, L., and Kety, S. S., "Regulation of cerebral circulation," Physiol. Rev. 40, Part II., Suppl. 4, p. 38 (1960).

368. Speransky, G. N., and Pratusevich, Yu. M., "On the rheoencephalographic correlates of acute mental tiredness in youngsters," Dokl. Akad. Nauk SSSR, 175:1193 (1967).

369. Sreseli, M. A., and Bol'shakov, O. P., "Structural features of the cavernous sinus and its role in regulation of the cerebral circulation," Transactions of the Institute of Experimental Morphology, Academy of Sciences of the Georgian SSR, Vol. 9. Tbilisi (1961), pp. 137-143.

370. Staub, N. C., "Microcirculation of the lung utilizing very rapid freezing," Angiology, 12:469 (1961).

371. Staudacher-Dalle Aste, E. V., and Rabito, C. S., "Ricerche anatomo-funzionali sulla regione del seno cavernoso umano," Boll. Soc. Ital. Biol. Sper., 16:589 (1941).

372. Stephens, W. E., "Discussion on vascular flow and turbulence," Neurology, 11(2):66 (1961).

373. Stöhr, P., "Die peripherische Nervenfaser," in: W. Möllendorf's Handbuch der Mikroskopischen Anatomie des Menschen, Vol. 4/1, Berlin (1928), pp. 143-201.

374. Stromberg, D. D., Shapiro, H. M., Lee, D. R., and Wiederheim, C. A., "Pial artery pressure in the cat, "in: 6th Conference on Microcirculation, Abstracts, Aalborg (1970), p. 172.

375. Sunzhas, M. U., "Surgical anatomy of the vertebral artery before entering the skull and its communication with the venous sinus," in: Disturbances of the Circulation in Brain Lesions, Moscow (1956), pp. 264-271.

376. Symon, L., "Observations on the leptomeningeal collateral circulation in dog," J. Physiol. (London), 154:1 (1960).

377. Symon, L., "An experimental study of traumatic cerebral vascular spasm," J. Neurol. Neurosurg. Psychiat., 30:497 (1967).

378. Symon, L., "A comparative study of middle cerebral pressure in dogs and macaques," J. Physiol. (London), 191:449 (1967).

379. Symon, L., Ishikawa, S., and Meyer, J., "Cerebral arterial pressure changes and development of leptomeningeal collateral circulation," Neurology, 13:237 (1963).

380. Tarasawa, F., "The experimental study on the nervous control of the cerebral circulation. I. The influences of stimulation of the cervical

sympathetic nerve on the blood flow in the internal and external carotid arteries. II. The influences of stimulation of the proximal end of the cut cervical vagal nerve on the tide arteries before and after cervical sympathectomy," Jap. Circulat. J., 25:1123 (1961).

381. Thuránszky, K., "Über die Rolle extra- und intraokularer Faktoren in der Regulation des Blutkreislaufs der Retina," Acta Physiol. Hung., 9:44 (1956).
382. Thuránszky, K., Der Blutkreislauf der Netzhaut., Budapest (1957).
383. Tkachenko, B. I., "Reflex changes in the cerebral circulation to stimulation of the coronary vessels," Fiziol. Zh. SSSR, 50:487 (1964).
384. Tkachev, R. A., Aleksandrova, L. I., and Prokhorova, E. S., "Hypertensive cerebral crises," in: Acute Disturbances of the Cerebral Circulation, Moscow (1960), pp. 35-43.
385. Torre, E. de la, Mitchell, O. C., and Netsky, M. G., "The seat of respiratory and cardiovascular responses to cerebral air emboli," Neurology, 12:140 (1962).
386. Torskaya, I. V., "Desquamation of epithelium of the capillaries as a cause of cerebral edema," Fiziol. Zh. (Ukr.), 6(5):669 (1960).
387. Tsuker, M., "Innervation of the chorioid plexus," Arch. Neurol. Psychiat. (Chicago), 58:474 (1947).
388. Tsvetkov, A. S., The Anatomy of Nerves of the Arteries at the Base of the Human Brain, Molotov (1948).
389. Ukolova, M. A., and Bordyushkov, Yu. N., "Linked changes in the blood supply to the brain and limb during sleep," Byull. Éksperim. Biol. i Med., 44(9):24 (1957).
390. Vamada, S., and Burton, A. C., "Effect of reduced tissue pressure on blood flow of the fingers; the veni-vasomotor reflex," J. Appl. Physiol., 6:501 (1954).
391. Van der Eecken, H. M., Anastomoses between the Leptomeningeal Arteries of the Brain. Their Morphology, Pathological and Clinical Significance, Thomas, Springfield (1959).
392. Vasadze, G. Sh., "Pathogenesis of severe traumatic and burn shock," in: Shock and Terminal States, Leningrad (1960), pp. 93-102.
393. Vasil'chenko, G. S., "Coagulation of the thalamo-tuberine artery for isolated occlusion of the blood supply to the anterior part of the thalamus in dogs," Vopr. Neirokhir., No. 4, p. 15 (1956).
394. Vasin, N. Ya., "Reflexes from the longitudinal sinus of the dura mater arising during sinusography," Fiziol. Zh. SSSR, 45:1201 (1959).
395. Vetrenko, T. V., "Reflexes from the meninges during application of mechanical stimuli," Vrach. Delo, No. 1, p. 11 (1957).
396. Voronin, V. V., Textbook of Pathological Physiology, Part 1, Tbilisi (1947).
397. Voronin, V. V., "The work of A. A. Bogomolets on the hemodynamics," Fiziol. Zh. (Ukr.), 11(3):29 (1956).
398. Wahl. M., Deetjen, P., Thurau, K., Ingvar, D. H., and Lassen, N. A., "Micropuncture evaluation of the importance of perivascular pH for the arteriolar diameter on the brain surface," Pflügers Arch. ges. Physiol. 316:152 (1970).
399. Waltz, A. G., "Effect of Pa_{CO_2} on blood flow and microcirculation of ischemic and nonischemic cerebral cortex," Stroke, 1:27 (1970).
400. Waltz, A. C., and Meyer, J. S., "Effects of change in composition of plasma on pial blood flow. II. High molecular weight substances, blood constituents and tonicity," Neurology, 9:815 (1959).
401. Waltz, A. G., and Sundt, T. M., "The microvasculature and microcirculation of the cerebral cortex after arterial occlusion," Brain, 90:681 (1967).
402. Waltz, A. G., and Sundt, T. M., "Influence of systemic blood pressure on blood flow and microcirculation of ischemic cerebral cortex," in: Luyendijk, W. (ed.), Progress in Brain Research, Vol. 30, Cerebral Circulation, Amsterdam (1968), pp. 107-112.
403. Wiśniewski, H., "Badania nad przepuszczalnoscia bariery: krew-mozg, krew–plyn mozgowo-rdzeniowy i plyn mozgowo-rdzeniowy–mozg dla bialek w warunkach fizjologicznych oraz bariery krew–mozg dla albumin w obrzeku mozgu" [Investigation of permeability of the blood–brain, blood–CSF, and CSF–brain barriers for protein under physiological conditions and of the blood–brain barrier for albumin in cerebral edema], Neuropatologia Polska, 3:1 (1965).
404. Wolff, H. G., and Forbes, H. S., "The cerebral circulation. V. Observations of the pial circulation during changes in intracranial pressure," Arch. Neurol. Psychiat. (Chicago), 20:1035 (1928).
405. Wyke, B., Brain Function and Metabolic Disorders, Butterworths, London (1963).

406. Yaure, G. G., "A special form of movement of fluid (blood) in healthy blood vessels," Dokl. Akad. Nauk SSSR, 56:919 (1947).

407. Yakhontov, V. I., "Material relating to active regulation of the blood vessels," Sborn. Nauchn. Trudov Stalingradsk. Med. Inst., 11:56 (1957).

408. Yoshida, K., Meyer, J. S., Sakamoto, K., and Handa, J., "Autoregulation of cerebral blood flow: electromagnetic flow measurements during acute hypertension in the monkey," Circulat. Res., 19:726 (1966).

409. Zaalishvili, I. M., "Rhythmic contractions of blood vessels," in: Collection of Papers to Commemorate 60 Years of V. V. Voronin's Scientific and Pedagogic Activities, Tbilisi (1952), pp. 103-108.

410. Zhitsa, V. T., "Contribution to the morphology of innervational mechanisms of cerebral arteries and veins," Arch. Anat. Gistol. i Émbriol., 58(1):27 (1970).

411. Zhukova, T. P., "The state of the vaso-capillary network of the cerebral hemispheres in animals of different ages during asphyxia. Report 2," Byull. Éksperim. Biol. i Med., 43(2):109 (1957).

412. Zilliacus, H., "The correlation between sedimentation rate and the intravascular aggregation of erythrocytes from the clinical aspect," Acta Med. Scand., 152:203 (1955).